ADORE YOURSELF SLIM

Eat, exercise and hypnotise yourself
to a healthier, happier you

Lisa Jackson

SIMON &
SCHUSTER

London · New York · Sydney · Toronto

A CBS COMPANY

To my mother Leoné Jackson,
who will always be an inspiration

Published in Great Britain by Simon & Schuster UK Ltd, 2011

A CBS Company

Simon and Schuster Illustrated Books
Simon & Schuster UK Ltd
222 Gray's Inn Road
London WC1X 8HB

1 2 3 4 5 6 7 8 9 10

Editorial director: Francine Lawrence
Design: Angela Ryan
Illustrations: Maxim Savva
Photography: Claire Richardson
Home economist for photography: Lizzie Harris
Stylist for photography: Prudence Ivey

Colour reproduction by Dot Gradations Ltd, UK
Printed and bound in China

ISBN 978-0-85720-162-1

SIMON &
SCHUSTER

CONTENTS

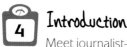

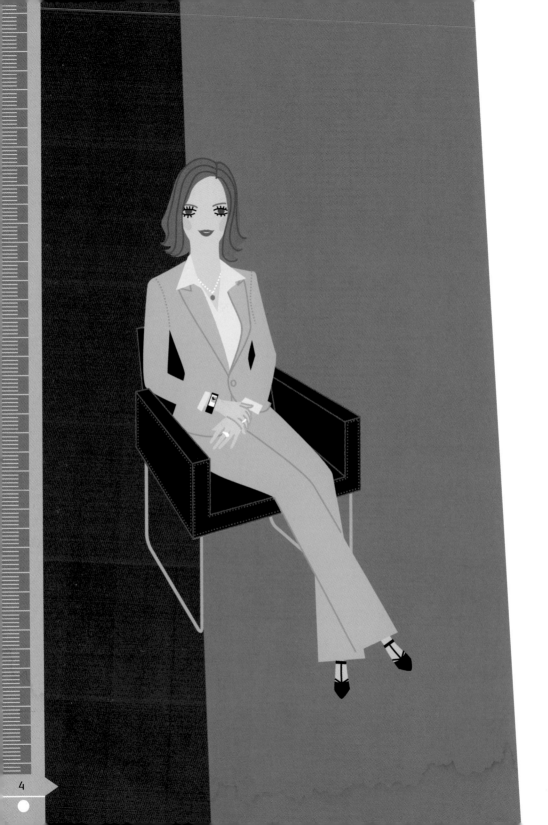

Introduction

Welcome to *Adore Yourself Slim*, a book that's designed to be your new best friend as you embark on the most exciting journey you'll ever make. By completing the fill-in sections you'll find throughout this book as you read it, you're going to create a remarkable record of every step you take towards becoming a slimmer, healthier, happier you. Because I've travelled my own weight-loss road, losing 3½st (22kg) along the way, I've personally tried and tested every single piece of expert eating, exercise and hypnosis advice this book contains. It's my privilege to join you on your journey. And once you reach your own Destination Dream Weight like I have, I truly wish that you, too, will be able to say that you thoroughly enjoyed the trip. Ready? Great, then let's set off…

Have you secretly lost hope of ever being able to lose weight? I know exactly how you're feeling. It wasn't that long ago that I was in the same situation, plagued by a weight problem that had dogged me virtually my entire adult life and despairing of ever being a healthy weight again. And yet here I am today, having found the courage to unpack the 3½st (22kg) of extra baggage I'd been carrying around with me every day for years.

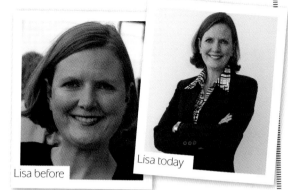

Lisa before

Lisa today

Along the way I discovered a lot about food, fitness and myself, and now I'd like to share everything I've learned with you. As a journalist-turned-hypnotherapist, I believe I'm in a unique position to do that. During the 11 years that I worked for a glossy women's health magazine, I gleaned loads of useful advice from the dozens of successful slimmers and experts I interviewed. And as the co-author of *Running Made Easy*, which is the UK's best-selling beginner's running book, I know a thing or two about motivation, inspiration – and perspiration! My new career as a certified clinical hypnotherapist has also convinced me that we have an enormously powerful tool at our disposal for changing our attitude towards our bodies, food and ourselves – our unconscious mind. Which is why this book comes with a five-track CD to enable you to overcome mental obstacles and set your sights firmly on success.

But most importantly, unlike the writers of other weight-loss books (most of whom have never even been remotely overweight), I've actually used all of the techniques in this book myself. I've cooked every recipe, sweated through every exercise, filled in the charts, practised self-hypnosis daily and rewarded myself for every single achievement. I'm living proof that it works.

This book is written to inspire you, to encourage you and to applaud you. It's designed to help you focus on the fabulous person you *already* are, as well as to help you transform yourself into an even better version of yourself. Today is the first day of the rest of your life. Isn't it time you began to adore yourself slim?

Lisa Jackson

THE START OF A GREAT LOVE AFFAIR

So what makes this book different from all the other weight-loss books you've got on your groaning bookshelf? Well, for a start, its primary focus is on self-esteem and self-belief, rather than calories in and calories out. Which is why I've called it *Adore Yourself Slim*. Over the following pages you're going to learn to truly appreciate yourself: in short, you're going to learn how to fall in love with yourself. And here's how this love affair – your new relationship with yourself – is going to unfold…

DITCH YOUR EMOTIONAL BAGGAGE

To succeed in a new relationship, you first have to make time to analyse what went wrong with your previous relationships, which is why the CD that accompanies this book contains a hypnosis track that will help you make peace with the past. Old diets that failed you, fitness plans you abandoned, unhealthy attitudes to food – it's time to learn from them and then consign them all to history so that you can move on.

LOVE AT FIRST SIGHT

When you picked up this book and saw how motivating and inspiring it looks compared with the host of dull and dreary weight-loss books out there, you may have felt an instant attraction. But remember, this is the start of a relationship with food, fitness and yourself that's going to last a lifetime. It's not a one-night stand, so we're not going to treat it like one. Which is why the eating plan isn't a short-term crash diet that gives you instant weight loss only to dash your hopes again when the pounds pile back on. It's healthy, realistic and designed to be doable long term. Just like the fitness plans.

SURVIVE A RELATIONSHIP CRISIS

All relationships go through rocky patches, and there'll inevitably be times when you reach a weight-loss plateau and start to wonder if things are really working. Overcoming this is key to long-term slimming success, which is why this book is packed with success-guaranteed hypnotic scripts, expert advice, quirky fitness ideas, crafty mental tricks and inspirational charts, graphs and journal pages for you to fill in, to get you back on track in no time.

CELEBRATE YOUR BIG DAY

Follow the psychological, eating and exercise advice in this book and, before you know it, it'll be time to celebrate getting to your goal weight – a day that's guaranteed to be almost as memorable (and photo worthy) as a wedding day. *Adore Yourself Slim* will be there with a glass of bubbly to celebrate, but will also give you easy strategies to make sure the weight stays off so that you can be certain this is a love affair for life – not just the honeymoon.

LOVE IS ALL YOU NEED

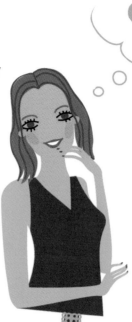

In this book you'll inevitably learn a lot about me – I'll share everything from my reasons for wanting to lose weight, to the tactics I used, to the compliments I got for doing so. But at the end of the day this isn't a book about me, it's about the most important person in your life – YOU!

So I'd like you now to pour yourself a glass of bubbly (or sparkling grape juice, if you must) and drink a toast to the incredible, wonderful, fabulously unique person you are. And while you're at it, take a few moments to list all the things you love about yourself, right here, right now. (Concentrate on what you love about your personality, as in Chapter 2 you'll get the chance to analyse what you love about your body.) Whether it's

66 Pour yourself a glass of bubbly (or sparkling grape juice) and drink a toast to the incredible, wonderful, fabulously unique person you are 99

the way you laugh, your generous nature or that you always say 'Thank you' to the bus driver when you alight from a bus – spend some time reflecting on and celebrating yourself. Looking sensational in a swimsuit may be a wonderful goal to strive towards, but if you don't already adore yourself right now for the person you really are, rather than the body you inhabit, you're definitely not going to be able to do so when you're slim.

Now spend some time seeing yourself as others see you and then write down everything your loved ones, friends and

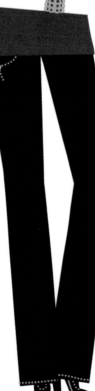

colleagues appreciate about you (if you get stuck, feel free to ask them – you may be wonderfully surprised to learn that what you take for granted they really rate). Whether it's the way you're always there when your friends need you, the sassy way you dress or the fact that you're the 'hostess with the mostest', get it all down on paper here.

Whenever you find it difficult sticking to this programme, or have one of those 'What's the point?' kind of days, turn back to these pages and read what you wrote to help rekindle your motivation.

10 THINGS I ADORE ABOUT MYSELF

1 _____

2 _____

3 _____

4 _____

5 _____

6 _____

7 _____

8 _____

9 _____

10 _____

10 THINGS OTHERS ADORE ABOUT ME

1 _____

2 _____

3 _____

4 _____

5 _____

6 _____

7 _____

8 _____

9 _____

10 _____

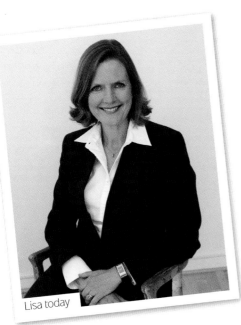
Lisa today

GET TO KNOW ME…

Before we really get started, I thought you might like to get to know me a little better first, and find out how I came to write *Adore Yourself Slim*…

My name is Lisa Jackson and I've been hungry almost my whole life. I have it on good authority that from the moment of my birth in a South African maternity hospital I started opening and closing my mouth like a goldfish, eager to be fed. By 12 I was the youngest member by about 20 years of a local slimming club, and yet at the time my weight problem was always something of a mystery to me, as we never had junk food at home. It's only now, looking back with the wisdom of hindsight, that I realise that my failure to eat breakfast and take a packed lunch to school would've wreaked havoc with my blood-sugar levels, leading me to binge on whatever I could get my hands on when I did eventually eat.

At university, toast-eating competitions made me gain more weight. After leaving university, I joined a slimming club (again) and made good progress, even though I hated weighing out all my food. Being spotted using the 'handy' fold-away scales by colleagues at the South African edition of *Cosmopolitan* magazine, where I'd started working as a sub-editor, was only fractionally less embarrassing than the very public weigh-ins at my weekly class, where the lecturer would always loudly enquire about where you were in your menstrual cycle if you'd gained a gram or two.

When I left South Africa, I unintentionally became the original Super Size Me! Long before Morgan Spurlock experimented with living off nothing but burgers for 30 days, I enjoyed a diet of the finest fast food morning, noon and night for 16 weeks – *four times* longer than he did! This unexpected experiment was conducted when, aged 24, I left South Africa with my husband Graham and went to Taiwan to teach English. The plan was to save up enough money to travel through South-East Asia for eight months before moving to the UK. I discovered that the most affordable food was to be found at roadside stalls. This food was healthy and tasty, but, never having travelled before, I was disconcerted to see that it was served on plates that only got the most cursory dunk in cold water before being used for the next customer. I soon decided I preferred eating my meals from sanitised polystyrene boxes in an air-conditioned restaurant, and so became a regular burger buyer. Photographs from this time reveal me ballooning into someone with cheeks so chubby I could have passed for a chipmunk.

Once I reached the UK, I became the couchiest of couch potatoes. I loathed exercise, and had a chronic aversion to walking that saw me driving to buy a pint of milk at the corner shop, which was all of a two-minute stroll away. My job at British *Cosmopolitan* magazine was very demanding and we often worked well after 9pm. I used this as an excuse to live on coffee, cigarettes and takeaways (often eaten standing up on the Tube home!).

Eventually I couldn't delude myself any longer. As I didn't have bathroom scales, I began to weigh myself at my local pharmacy. I watched in morbid fascination as month by month the scales printed out little slips of paper chronicling my weight gain. Despairing, I rejoined a slimming club. I lost the same 4lb (1.8kg) three times before conceding that it just wasn't going to work for me this time.

Lisa before

At the age of 29, I started working at a health magazine where everyone seemed to walk around clutching a bottle of mineral water. After just a few weeks I'd succumbed to this subtle form of peer pressure and I, too, began drinking water and taking seven loo breaks a day instead of seven fag breaks. I also discovered a hidden passion for running that saw me complete a three-mile (5km) race and the London Marathon ten months later. But despite these lifestyle changes my weight remained stubbornly high, so I embarked on a series of unsuccessful fad diets that never lasted more than a couple of days or weeks.

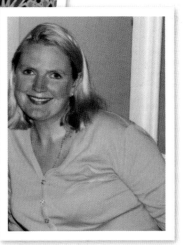

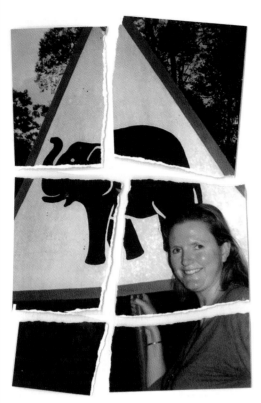

displayed in its full glory. The photo was such a graphic reminder of how overweight I'd become that I tore it up and continued to hurriedly edit the rest. So engrossed was I in this task that I failed to notice that Graham had absent-mindedly pieced together all the torn-up pieces of the photo, like a jigsaw puzzle, and that our guests were now casting sneaky glances at it to find out why I'd made such a big fuss. I appeared to simply laugh it off, but deep down I was mortified. All the same, I just couldn't find it in myself to pluck up the courage to go on yet another diet.

When I later co-wrote a beginner's running book called *Running Made Easy*, almost everyone I interviewed mentioned how running had helped them lose weight. And yet, six years after I'd first donned my trainers, and despite having completed numerous marathons (very, very slowly) by that time, I still hadn't managed to lose any of the weight I'd put on. I was dreading the book launch when I'd have to come face to face with the reading public. What bothered me most wasn't the fact that I wasn't super-slim, it was the fact that I was an unhealthy weight and wasn't a good role model for my readers. I kept wishing fervently that the blessed BMI (body mass index) chart had never been invented.

When you're overweight, you feel that cameras should have to pass a lie-detector test, as they always seem to lie! Whenever I saw photos of myself I'd always be furious at the way they seemed to make me look enormous (and often blamed the photographer!). One summer, when we were hosting a barbecue, Graham brought out our recent holiday photos to show our friends. As always, I snatched them before they were passed round to censor them and, as I shuffled through the pile, I spotted a particularly hideous picture of myself posing in front of a sign at Angkor Wat in Cambodia warning motorists to beware of elephants crossing the road (above). Red-faced and sweaty, each of my numerous double chins was

A chance conversation in our office kitchen changed my life for ever. My colleague Jenny, who had recently lost a lot of weight, mentioned that she was following a low-carb diet. By this time I'd just about given up on ever being able to lose weight again, but that very day I went out and bought the book she recommended. However, I was disappointed to see that it involved eating a range of different cooked breakfasts and was packed with fiddly-looking recipes. My morning routine barely allowed time for brushing my teeth, let alone concocting cunning little frittatas in a muffin tin before work. And so the book lay forgotten for a month or so as the date of the launch of *Running Made Easy* loomed ever closer.

Everyone needs a good nag every so often. And Jenny did just that a month later when she enquired whether I'd been following the diet. When I explained my reasons for not attempting it, she simply refused to let me get away with my lame excuses and told me to combine the second phase of the plan, where you're allowed to have oats for breakfast, with the first, more rigidly low-carb phase. She also advised me to ditch the recipes and just cook items off the list of

> ## 66 By combining hypnosis and healthy eating with running and resistance training I lost just over 2½st (16.3kg) in only two-and-a-half months 99

permissible foods in any way I liked. I did as she suggested, and having made several other adaptations to the plan, was delighted when I lost 4lb (1.8kg) in the first week.

At about this time, my physiotherapist suggested I contact Coach Bronek, a Polish fitness trainer, whom she said would help me shed the weight that was causing my recurring running injuries. I warmed to him immediately, even though I was close to tears when he asked me

to do lunges with handweights and I only managed five. I could only afford to see him once a week for six weeks – after that I only saw him once every two months. But in the interim I religiously followed his training programmes two to three times a week and was amazed by the results. Each session was super-tough, but when I emerged from the gym with my hair so wet with sweat that it looked as if I'd been swimming, I knew that I'd made the most of every one of those 60 minutes. And before too long I was doing an astonishing 120 lunges with ease.

By now I'd started to dare to hope that I could lose weight, and so I decided to go the whole hog and sign up for a six-week course of hypnotherapy, too. The hypnosis sessions taught me to prioritise my health and totally changed my relationship with food: instead of automatically raiding the fridge in search of a food-fix, I learned to listen to my body and hear whether it was asking for food, an early night or a hug. By combining hypnosis and healthy eating with running and resistance training, I lost just over 2½st (16.3kg) in only two-and-a-half months. I'll never forget the comedy moment when my trousers became so loose that they almost fell to my ankles as I walked to work one morning. Nor will I forget the book launch where I was able to address the assembled throng with my head held high.

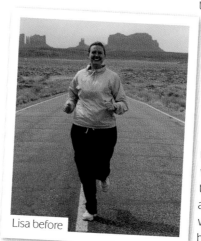
Lisa before

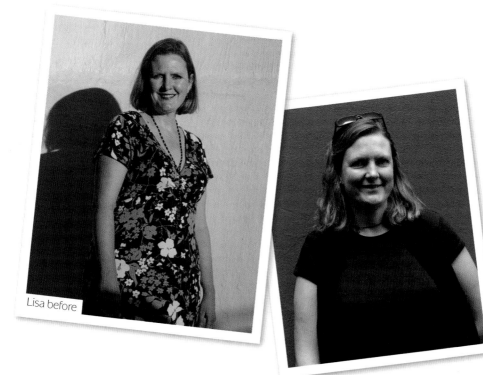

Lisa before

Ironically, everything (including my figure) went pear-shaped when I decided to train as a clinical hypnotherapist. I began spending up to five hours a day studying, on top of a demanding day job and a two-hour daily commute. And despite the fact that my course continued to convince me of the incredible benefits of hypnosis, I skipped my self-hypnosis sessions and used the time to cram in more study. In an attempt to keep my energy levels up, I abandoned my eating plan and began to eat virtually from the moment I got up to the minute before I crashed into bed each night. And whereas before I'd gone to the gym at lunchtimes and run part of the way home, I now began to revise in my lunch-hour and caught the bus home instead so that I could squeeze in an extra 20 minutes of revision. I was delighted

when I gained my diploma – but less delighted by the pounds I'd put back on along the way. When I came to do my post-graduate diploma in hypnotherapy, the same thing happened and I put on even more weight.

It was when my underwear started to cut into me like cheesewire that I knew it was time to take control of my weight again. When I'd slimmed down before, I'd weighed myself every day and had found this a very motivating way to stay on track. However, my scales had been gathering dust during the time it took me to qualify as a hypnotherapist. When I stepped on them for the first time in two years, I couldn't believe my eyes. At just under 14st (88.3kg) I was heavier than I'd ever been in my whole life. And if that wasn't bad enough, the BMI chart in my running book said that my BMI of 30.6 meant that I was now officially heavy enough to be classified as 'obese'. I stepped off the scales feeling as if I'd entered a parallel universe – I couldn't possibly be obese! I'd run *marathons* for goodness sake!

'Goals are dreams with deadlines' is one of my favourite quotes, so I set about deciding on a deadline for my weight-loss goal. Graham was going to Bangladesh for a three-month secondment, but was due to come home for a long weekend after six weeks, so I used that as my first deadline. The day after he left, I began to set everything in place to make sure that this time I would definitely succeed in reaching my goal. What made it easier was knowing

> 66 **Every time I was tempted to obsess about my marshmallow thighs, I gave myself a really stern talking to and focused on my swan-like neck instead** 99

that I definitely knew how to do it – I had a plan that I knew couldn't fail. I decided to take a three-pronged approach and use everything I'd found useful in my hypnotherapy courses, all that Coach Bronek had taught me plus everything I'd ever learned while working on the health magazine to create a way of life that would enable me to lose weight – and keep it off – for good.

The first thing I did was analyse what had gone wrong before. I realised exercise, on its own, wasn't the answer. Nor was being very knowledgeable about hypnosis – but not actually practising it! I also concluded that I couldn't simply eat whatever I liked just because I was exercising.

Next I drew up a list of the reasons why I wanted to be slim, followed by a list of why I already loved myself (lumps, bumps and all), as I knew that self-love and not self-loathing would be key to my success. I then promised myself a series of treats to celebrate every weight-loss milestone and enlisted my Canadian friend Bridget Robinson as my slimming buddy. I began practising self-hypnosis on the train to work in the mornings. And I dusted off Coach Bronek's resistance-training programmes. I also began doing ten squats, lunges or wall press-ups whenever I got the chance and started doing speed training and hill training with my colleagues twice a week. And every single time I was tempted to obsess about my marshmallow thighs, I gave myself a really stern talking to and focused on my swan-like neck and twig-like wrists for a few seconds instead.

As for my eating plan, I wanted to make sure that all of the new habits I'd adopted complied with current best-practice advice on healthy eating, and so could be followed permanently. That's why I decided to ask Lyndel Costain, a leading dietitian, whom I'd come to know through editing her articles for the health magazine I worked on, to take a look at the eating plan I'd devised and suggest ways to make it even more healthy, effective and doable. I was thrilled when Lyndel told me that my plan was fundamentally sound and would need only a few tweaks to ensure it offered all the health benefits I felt were so vital. Knowing I was accountable to her also made a big difference (my husband's new motto whenever I was tempted to order a takeaway became: 'What would Lyndel say?').

And so the *Adore Yourself Slim* Eating Plan was born. This time I lost 1½st (9.5kg) in just two months, and the compliments, which I took delight in recording in my Filofax, came flooding in. But I also went through periods when life got in the way. My beloved mum was tragically killed in an accident and suddenly weight loss was the last thing on my mind. I plateaued and lost hope, but found it again when I came to realise that nothing would've made my mum happier or more proud than for me to pick myself up, dust myself down and continue with my weight-loss journey.

The result is this book, which contains all the strategies I've used to help me lose 3½st (22kg) in total. I've lived and breathed this book, so it isn't just a collection of expert wisdom or unrealistic advice – it's a compilation of every single thing I did that worked and that I know will also work for you. Everything's designed to be affordable and fit into a hectic lifestyle, because, like you, I don't have endless cash to splash or time to spare. I know this book will help you to achieve your weight-loss goals, too, and that you'll be able to say, hand on heart, that you've loved every minute of this grand adventure.

> 66 **I've lived and breathed this book – it's a compilation of every single thing I did that worked and that I know will also work for you** 99

Lisa now

YOUR STORY IN YOUR OWN WORDS

Now that I've shared my story with you, it's time to make a start on your own success story. On the pages overleaf there's space for you to chart your very own weight-loss odyssey. Every few weeks or so, come back to these pages and reflect on your triumphs, your challenges and how far you've come, before filling in the relevant sections. One day, and it's sooner than you might think, your story will be complete and you'll be at Destination Dream Weight, toasting your success with a glass of bubbly and looking forward to living happily and healthily ever after!

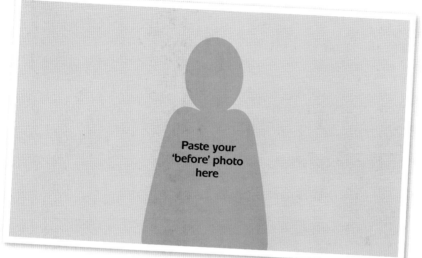

Paste your 'before' photo here

Me before (date)

_____

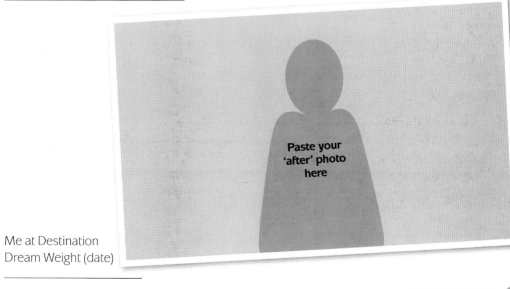

Paste your 'after' photo here

Me at Destination Dream Weight (date)

_____

THE SECRET OF MY SUCCESS

MY PAST (BEFORE I EMBARKED ON MY *ADORE YOURSELF SLIM* JOURNEY)

I was a slim/slightly chubby/overweight child/teenager because

_____

_____

I gained weight because

_____

_____

_____

_____

When I realised I was overweight, I felt the following about myself

_____

_____

_____

_____

I reached my heaviest weight at the age of _____. At that time my diet consisted of
Breakfast _____

_____

Lunch _____

_____

Dinner _____

_____

Drinks/snacks _____

_____

_____

MY *ADORE YOURSELF SLIM* JOURNEY

The turning point came on _____ (date) when I decided to lose weight for good and adore myself slim.

The three main reasons I wanted to be slimmer were

1 _____

2 _____

3 _____

When I read *Adore Yourself Slim*, I decided it could work for me because

_____

_____

_____

_____

What I loved about the plan was

_____

_____

_____

What I found most challenging about following the plan was

_____

_____

_____

> **❝ You gain strength, courage and confidence by every experience in which you really stop to look fear in the face... You must do the thing which you think you cannot do ❞**
> *US First Lady Eleanor Roosevelt*

When I lost my first ½st (3.2kg), I rewarded myself with

and I felt

Whenever I listened to the hypnosis CD, I felt

The biggest mistakes I made when following the plan were (optional)

1

2

3

But I rectified them by adopting the following strategies

1

2

3

My friends and family reacted to the newly slim me by

My favourite compliments were

Now I eat the following in a typical day
Breakfast

Snack

Lunch

Snack

Dinner

Drinks

I know I can maintain this weight because

When I drank my first glass of bubbly/my favourite tipple before starting the plan, I felt

When I celebrated reaching Destination Dream Weight with a glass of bubbly/my favourite tipple, I felt

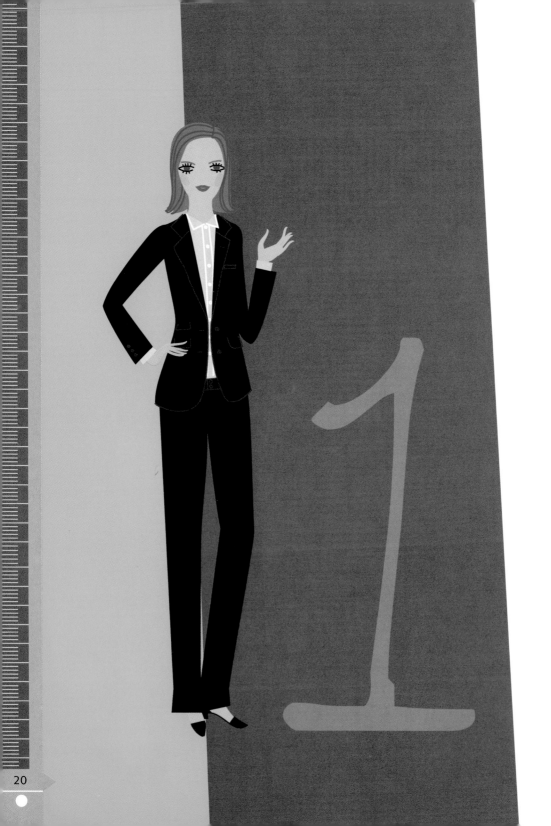

Chapter 1

THINK
yourself
SLIM

Just because diets and other weight-loss programmes have failed you before doesn't mean you have to resign yourself to a body you're less than happy with. By helping you discover the real reasons you've gained those unwanted pounds and encouraging you to make peace with the past using hypnosis, this chapter will become your first step in the breathtakingly exciting adventure that you'll one day look back on as the time that you, finally, started adoring yourself slim…

MAKE PEACE WITH THE PAST

Before we plunge headlong into the *Adore Yourself Slim* eating and exercise plan, let's take a few minutes to revisit the past and analyse how and why those pounds crept on in the first place and/or why you're struggling to lose weight now. Once you know the answers to these questions, you can use the information to make sure you succeed in getting to, and staying at, your goal weight, because you'll be more aware of the habits and lifestyle choices that have been unhelpful.

In the first section, top right, list the factors that have contributed to your weight gain. Or, if it's more helpful, think of this in terms of what's been getting in the way of you losing weight. Look closely at the following:
a) your attitude to exercise (for example, 'I'm not sporty' or 'I find exercising boring')
b) your eating habits (for example, 'I skip breakfast and have a serious cupcake habit')
c) your family commitments (for example, 'I'm so busy looking after my kids that I don't have time to cook healthy meals')
d) your leisure pursuits (for example, 'I watch 42 hours of television a week')
e) your working day (for example, 'I eat at my desk – and often visit the vending machine')

Next I'd like you to analyse the emotional reasons you may have had for becoming overweight (or that have been making it hard for you to lose weight). Have you been prescribing yourself fattening food in an attempt to comfort yourself when you've felt unloved or unhappy, for instance? Do you eat out of boredom or anger? Or because you're feeling exhausted or frustrated? Or do you eat what you consider a 'bad' food and then feel that you've failed and so keep on eating? Look closely at the following:
a) your emotions (for example, 'I comfort eat whenever I'm stressed')
b) your view of yourself (for example, 'I don't actually like myself enough to make an effort to lose weight')
c) your relationships with your parents, partner, friends and family (for example, 'My parents taught me to always finish all the food on my plate')

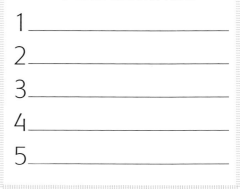

5 REASONS WHY MY LIFESTYLE LED TO WEIGHT GAIN/MAKES IT HARD TO LOSE WEIGHT NOW

1 _____

2 _____

3 _____

4 _____

5 _____

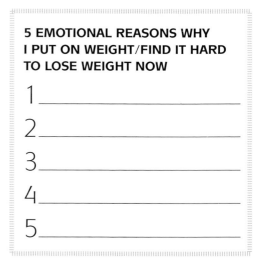

5 EMOTIONAL REASONS WHY I PUT ON WEIGHT/FIND IT HARD TO LOSE WEIGHT NOW

1 _____

2 _____

3 _____

4 _____

5 _____

HYPNOSIS: YOUR SECRET SLIMMING TOOL

Adore Yourself Slim is unique in that it not only features detailed expert eating and exercise plans but also harnesses an incredibly powerful tool: your unconscious mind. By using the five hypnosis tracks (which I call your Secret Slimming Tools) that I've recorded for you on the CD that accompanies this book, you're going to learn how to give your motivation and willpower a huge boost.

Numerous studies have been conducted into the benefits of using hypnosis for weight loss – and the results are encouraging. In one study[1], the hypnosis group lost an average of 1st 3lb (7.7kg) in six months, whereas the non-hypnosis group, which followed the same weight-management programme, lost only ½lb (0.22kg).

The long-term effects of using hypnosis for weight loss were also demonstrated in another study[2], published in the *Journal of Clinical Psychology*, in which 109 overweight people were put on a medically supervised weight-loss programme, some of whom were given hypnotherapy regularly while others weren't. Both groups lost weight, but interestingly, whereas the hypnosis group continued to lose weight up to and including the two-year follow-up, the non-hypnosis group either stopped losing weight or regained most of it after two years.

It's important to remember, though, that hypnosis is not a magic wand (even though we'd all secretly like it to be!). Rather, it's a tool to help enable behaviour change. While listening to the CD will undoubtedly make it easier for you to lose weight and reduce your stress levels, it doesn't mean you can continue with the unhelpful eating and exercise patterns that made you gain weight in the first place. You need to take a conscious decision to change first, and then my hypnosis tracks will help you to stay focused and enthusiastic about implementing those changes to ensure they remain a permanent fixture in your life.

SO HOW EXACTLY DOES IT WORK?

Hypnosis is a state of deep physical relaxation that allows your conscious mind to 'get out of the way', thereby allowing you to communicate directly with your unconscious mind, which is where all the information that influences your actions is stored. When you're in this focused mental state, you're better able to accept beneficial, life-changing suggestions, which, if you were in a waking state, you might reject (or talk yourself out of!). By replacing your deep-seated negative beliefs ('I'm not sporty', 'I always comfort eat when I'm unhappy' – see the lists you drew up on the opposite page) with positive beliefs ('I embrace exercise because it makes me feel amazing', 'I eat only when I'm truly hungry'), hypnosis can help you to achieve the weight-loss goals you've set yourself. Imagining yourself performing all the new, healthier habits a slimmer version of you would have acquired also helps to ingrain these actions, so that when you're no longer in a hypnotic state you're more likely to carry them out in everyday life.

HYPNOSIS DEMYSTIFIED

If you're apprehensive about using hypnosis as your Secret Slimming Tool, then you're not alone. When many people think of hypnosis, the first image that springs to mind is stage hypnosis – where members of the audience generally embarrass themselves in public. Stage hypnotists usually select subjects who are extrovert and enjoy having a laugh. For the participants in a stage show, there is also an element of peer pressure (they may not want to be the only person up on stage not amusing the crowd with their outrageous antics) and the alcohol factor (participants will probably have had a drink or two before the show starts, which will have helped to lower their inhibitions). And, of course, if the participants do end up doing embarrassing things, then they can always blame the hypnotist and say that he or she 'made' them do it!

The kind of clinical hypnotherapy you'll be experiencing when you practise self-hypnosis (see page 44) and listen to the CD is completely different. When you experience hypnotherapy for yourself, you'll see that you simply sit in a quiet place and allow yourself to become very relaxed – at no time will you start behaving like a chicken or do anything that could be considered remotely entertaining or embarrassing.

YOU'RE IN CONTROL

All hypnosis is self-hypnosis – a hypnotherapist's voice is just one way to help you reach the state of deep relaxation we call a hypnotic state. It's easier and quicker if someone else guides you into it, which is why I've included a CD with this book, but most people are perfectly capable of hypnotising themselves once they know how. To help prove this point, I've included a self-hypnosis session on page 44 (to help you analyse your real reasons for wanting to lose weight). It's important to remember that you remain in control throughout every hypnosis session, and if you ever want the session to end, all you need do is open your eyes and you'll return to waking consciousness. It's a movie-inspired myth that you can get 'stuck' in hypnosis. If the hypnotherapist doesn't formally awaken you, all that would happen is that you would remain relaxed until you either fell asleep, felt ready to wake up or became hungry.

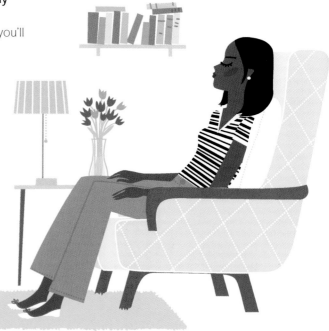

YOU CAN'T BE FORCED TO DO THINGS

My voice (or any other hypnotherapist's voice, for that matter) can't 'force' you to do anything because hypnosis doesn't work like that. Before you decide to allow yourself to be hypnotised, you need to have made a conscious decision that you actually want to make the changes that the hypnotherapist is going to suggest to you. By buying this book you've already indicated your willingness to change – and the hypnosis CD is simply going to reinforce that. Your unconscious mind has an incredible defence mechanism that prevents negative suggestions, or suggestions that might go against your moral beliefs, being accepted. Were you to hear such a suggestion, you would simply bring

> **❝ Once you've made the decision to change, the hypnotic state makes positive suggestions more likely to influence your actions when you're awake ❞**

yourself out of hypnosis, as the heightened state of awareness you're in during hypnosis enables you to both reject and accept suggestions, as you would when fully awake. However, this state also makes positive suggestions more likely to take hold and influence your actions when you're awake. And that's why listening to all my brilliant suggestions on the CD will help to bring you ever closer to Destination Dream Weight.

WHAT HYPNOSIS FEELS LIKE

What many people don't realise is that we frequently experience hypnotic states in everyday life. When you become so deeply engrossed in a book that you don't notice the phone's ringing, or when you drive a familiar route, arrive at your destination and can't remember how you got there, you've been in a hypnotic state – your conscious mind has switched off and you've been functioning on autopilot. Daydreaming is another example of being in a hypnotic state.

Everyone experiences hypnosis differently. When you listen to the CD that accompanies this book, at times you may think that you can remember every word, whereas at other times you may feel that you've drifted away and not heard most of what I've said. On yet other occasions, you may recall some sections of a track and not others. Rest assured that whatever you experience is normal and doesn't mean you haven't been hypnotised. As long as you're relaxed, your unconscious mind will remember everything that it's important for you to remember.

If you're looking for tangible evidence that you have indeed entered a hypnotic state, then you could try timing your hypnosis session. Time distortion (along with feeling that you're less aware of your body and your surroundings) is a commonly occurring hypnotic phenomenon and you may be surprised to find that what you thought was a 30-minute session actually only lasted 10 minutes, or that 10 minutes feels as if it has passed by really slowly. Other hypnotic phenomena that may occur are feeling that you're drifting or floating, experiencing tingling, heaviness or numbness in your hands and legs or even feeling that you can't move your limbs. These sensations are actually very pleasurable (they're like that wonderful Sunday-morning lie-in feeling where you know you can get up, but are so relaxed that you can't be bothered to), and aren't cause for concern. If you did want to move for any reason, then simply opening your eyes would end the session and enable you to do so.

PRACTICE MAKES PERFECT

Hypnosis works best with constant repetition. Just as a jungle path will soon turn into a road if it's used often enough, so too will your new positive beliefs become stronger, and more habitual, the more often you think them. Similarly, just as a jungle path will soon grow over if it's never used, so your negative beliefs will become weaker the less often you think them. Just think of a memory from your childhood. You may have been only two when a very cheeky duck stole a biscuit out of your hand in the park (as one memorably did to me!), but if your parents repeatedly reminded you of that story, you're likely to be able to remember it until you're 90. If, however, that incident was never mentioned again, that memory would have slowly faded and you would be unlikely to be able to recall it now.

PUT ON YOUR GOAL GLASSES

Because repetition is so vital to the success of hypnosis, after you've listened to Track 1 a few times, in Chapters 4 and 5 I'm going to ask you to start listening to Tracks 2 and 3 twice a day, once in the morning and once in the evening. These tracks will not only help to change your self-limiting beliefs but will also help to remind you of what you're trying to achieve. While some people find it more difficult than others to lose weight (due to, for example, genetic differences in appetite or a medical problem), successful weight loss is largely a matter of choice. First you decide to shed those unwanted pounds, and then you go about making hundreds of tiny choices, day in, day out, that will either help you to succeed – or derail your efforts. It's helpful to think of your twice-daily

> 66 As a single footstep will not make a path on the earth, so a single thought will not make a pathway in the mind. To make a deep physical path, we walk again and again. To make a deep mental path, we must think over and over the kind of thoughts we wish to dominate our lives 99
> **Henry David Thoreau**

HYPNOTISE YOURSELF SLIM: TRACK 1

Now it's time to experience hypnosis for yourself and let go of everything that's been preventing your weight loss until now. Find a quiet place where you won't be disturbed, make yourself comfortable (be sure you've gone to the loo first and are warm enough), sit back, relax and listen to Track 1 (Make Peace With The Past) on your hypnosis CD. At the end of this 20-minute hypnosis session you'll have put the past behind you and be ready to start making the positive changes to your lifestyle that will help you adore yourself slim. If you have a lot of issues you want to deal with, you may choose to listen to this track a few times to ensure that you've covered everything before you move on.

---

hypnosis sessions as putting on a pair of what I call Goal Glasses with the words 'I adore myself slim' etched on the inside of them. These Goal Glasses will enable you to go about your everyday life as normal, but each and every time you're faced with a choice (whether to cave in and have that slab of cheesecake or not go for a walk, for example), seeing those words in front of you will remind you of what you've set out to do and reinforce your desire to make the positive choice that will be a step forwards on your weight-loss journey, rather than a step backwards. When you practise hypnosis last thing at night, it'll send a powerful message to your unconscious mind that reaching your goal is vitally important to you, and those thoughts will be laid down as new beliefs in your unconscious mind while you sleep.

▶ CAN EVERYONE BE HYPNOTISED?

The general rule is that if you really want to be hypnotised, you can be. By the same token, you can't be hypnotised against your will. Hypnosis is not recommended for people suffering from psychotic conditions, such as schizophrenia, as the dissociation you may experience during hypnosis (feelings of being unaware of time, your body or your surroundings) can aggravate your illness. If you're in any doubt as to whether you're a suitable candidate for hypnosis, first consult your GP. It is also important to avoid going into a hypnotic state if you are under the influence of alcohol or recreational drugs. These substances create artificial states of altered awareness that are incompatible with the therapeutic hypnotic state. By combining the two states, you would either fall asleep or find that your mind was unable to respond coherently to the suggestions being given.

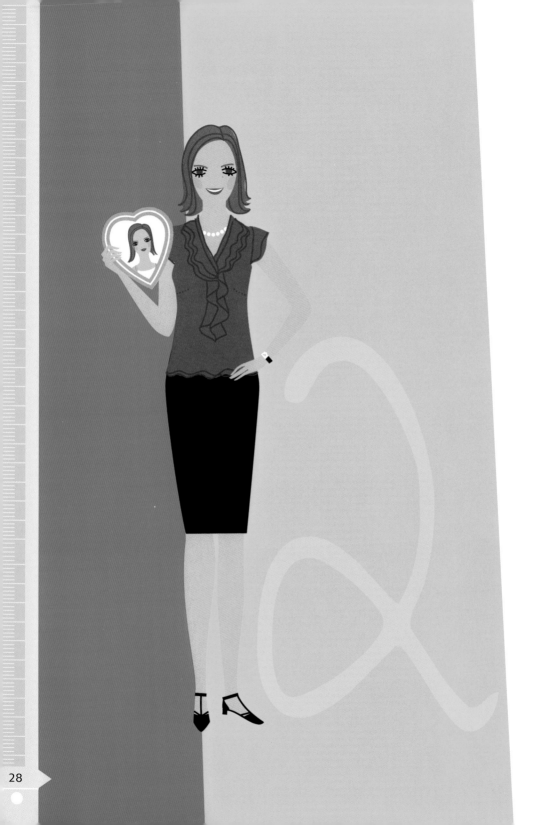

Chapter 2

Learn to ADORE yourself SLIM

Now that you've made peace with the past, it's time to look to the future and develop the strategies, skills and survival tactics that will take you all the way to slimming success. To ensure that you stay motivated, I've also included case histories and real-life stories from women just like you who dared to decide to be slimmer, and who are now loving life more than ever…

THE *ADORE YOURSELF SLIM* BODY SCAN

How are you feeling? When I ask this question, I'm not expecting the typically unthinking response, 'Fine, thanks.' I'm asking you to take a long, hard look at yourself and tell me how you're *really* feeling. Deep down, in the very fibre of your being. When I was living on nicotine and caffeine and doing no exercise, my answer would have been: 'Slightly nauseous, exhausted and edgy.' Ask me that same question today, and I'm more likely to reply: 'Enthusiastic, energised and wonderful.' Because that's the effect that taking care of your body has on you – everything, simply everything, looks and feels a little better when you're exercising and eating well.

However, when you're slimming, it can be easy to forget how downright great being lighter and eating more healthily makes you feel. Losing weight isn't just about shedding pounds, it's about feeling better about life, the universe – everything! So I'd like you to set aside a few minutes now to complete a simple Body Scan. Don't worry if you're claustrophobic – this doesn't involve high-tech equipment, just the ability to concentrate.

▶ HOW TO PERFORM A BODY SCAN

Step 1 Make yourself comfortable by either sitting in a chair or lying down, and close your eyes. Focus on your breathing for a few moments, to clear your mind.

Step 2 Turn your attention inwards and start to scan your body, imagining a laser beam sweeping slowly downwards, from your head to your toes, that allows you to become aware of how each part of your body feels. When you scan your head, do you feel bright, alert, positive and optimistic? When you scan your chest, do your lungs feel healthy or are you wheezing slightly? When you scan your stomach, do you feel that the food you've been eating has made you feel satisfied but not stuffed; healthy and energised rather than sluggish and lethargic? When you scan your fingertips and toes, do they feel truly alive or do you have difficulty imagining that they're actually part of your body? Next assess your energy levels. Are you brimming with enthusiasm and raring to go, or do you feel tired, which is how you feel much of the time?

Step 3 When you've finished doing your Body Scan, spend a few more moments analysing exactly how you feel in your body generally. Do you feel comfortable, content, happy and energetic, or do you feel uncomfortable, dissatisfied, unhappy and apathetic? Now create a snapshot of exactly how you feel today and write down your findings here:

■ At the start of my weight-loss journey, this is the way I feel about my body/the way I'm currently living my life

_____
_____
_____

■ This is what I'd prefer to feel about my body and the way I live my life

_____
_____
_____
_____

I devised this Body Scan exercise for my patients because of an experience I had when I visited Amsterdam for a long weekend with my husband Graham and sister-in-law Deb several years ago. Having eaten healthily for several months, I was really looking forward to letting my hair down and treating myself to foods that I wouldn't usually eat, such as the local speciality *Vlaamse frites* (chips with mayonnaise). And so we

> **❝ My body was in open revolt – it was crying out for healthy food, and although the 'naughty' fatty food had tasted quite good at the time (though it wasn't nearly as tasty as I thought it would be!), it left me feeling dreadful ❞**

started our three-day break with me steadfastly refusing the fruit salad breakfast the others opted for and instead insisting on a croissant. After lunching on baguettes and eating the famous *Vlaamse frites* for dinner, I woke up the next day feeling terrible, but still insisted on the croissant I'd promised myself instead of the more virtuous fruit salad and muesli my husband and Deb chose to have.

By dinnertime that day, however, I had to concede defeat. My body was in revolt – it was crying out for healthy food, and although the 'naughty' fatty food tasted quite good (to be honest, it wasn't nearly as tasty as I thought it would be!), it left me feeling dreadful. Instead of waking up feeling energetic and raring to go, I felt bloated, sluggish and slightly nauseous. I realised then and there that, while my weight wouldn't be sabotaged by just one mini-break of fat-laden indulgence, I'd reprogrammed my body to insist on wholesome food and it wasn't prepared to go back to its old ways.

Now, years later, whenever I find myself going through a 'Bloody heck, I'm tired of being good' phase, I call up that image of myself feeling really unwell, and it's enough to get me back on the straight and narrow in an instant.

■ At the moment, I'm unable to do the following because of my weight (eg walk up a flight of stairs without becoming breathless; wear a bikini)

_____

_____

_____

■ When I've reached my Destination Dream Weight, I'd like to be able to do the following (eg wear jeans again; run a three-mile/5km race; love clothes shopping)

_____

_____

Step 4 Now I'd like you to store that image of yourself at your current weight somewhere in your unconscious mind, so that when you've adopted healthier habits but are tempted to revert to your old ways, you'll be able to compare your new, more lively, more positive self to your less energetic, less positive 'old' self. Being reminded of how uncomfortable or sluggish you felt at the start of this programme will help to convince you to persevere.

HOW TO DEVELOP UNSHAKEABLE SELF-BELIEF

You're just about to embark on a very exciting journey, but be warned – like any adventure there are bound to be highs ('Hoorah, just look what the scales say' days) and lows ('Boy, do I have a long, long way to go' moments) along the road. Staying upbeat in the months that lie ahead isn't always going to be easy, so I've come up with a few suggestions to help you keep your self-belief sky high. Work out ways to incorporate them into your everyday life to make sure that this time you'll adore (not 'abhor' or 'deplore') yourself slim…

Take a daily Praise Pill. One of the most inspiring, no-nonsense self-help books I've read in a long time is *Life's Too F***ing Short* by Janet Street-Porter. One line in particular had me laughing out loud, until I realised the hidden truth in it: 'Spend the first minute of every day telling yourself "I am bloody brilliant" – no one else is going to!' Though I don't agree with the last bit (during my own weight-loss journey I was touched by how many of my family, friends and colleagues expressed admiration for what I was doing), we should all spend the first precious minute of every morning praising and encouraging ourselves. That way, even if no one else does, it doesn't matter, we've taken our Praise Pill for the day.

Stop striving to be perfect. It's time we realised that there really isn't a universal image of perfection that we must attain in order for us to love ourselves and be loved by others. One way to stop berating ourselves constantly for not living up to this unrealistic ideal is to start practising unconditional self-acceptance. Repeat to yourself as often as you can: 'I am a fallible, unique, worthwhile human being'. And stop beating yourself up about mistakes (that workout you skipped, that secret trip to the vending machine) – just vow to learn from them and write your insights in your *Adore Yourself Slim* Travel Journal on page 148.

Get in touch with your body. Show your body just how much you adore it by lavishing it with care and attention. Applying a scented body lotion is a fantastic way to connect with your body and send it a message that you love it for what it can do (carry you around, give you sensual pleasure, allow you to enjoy all the wonderful things life has to offer), not just for the way it looks.

Evict the Wicked Witch. It's believed that we have an incredible 10,000 thoughts a day, but have you ever stopped to think how many of them are negative? Tune in to the little voice in your head and you may be surprised to find how instead of a Fairy Godmother bestowing blessings on your life you've got the Wicked Witch of the West belittling, criticising and sneering at everything you do. Fortunately, there's a simple way to evict the Wicked Witch: whenever you catch yourself thinking something that's unhelpful ('I'll always be overweight'), imagine a giant STOP sign springing up in front of your face and someone holding a megaphone bellowing 'STOP' at you. Then consciously and deliberately turn that thought into a positive ('Every day, in every way, I'm becoming slimmer and fitter') and watch that Wicked Witch and her Flying Monkeys flee.

Make 'love' the most over-used word in your vocabulary. Journalist Lesley Garner, the author of one of my favourite-ever mood-boosting books, *Everything I've Ever Done That Worked*, is a firm believer, as am I, of William Morris's adage that we should not have anything in our homes that we don't know to be useful or believe to be beautiful. The same goes for your life. Take a long, hard look at every aspect of your life and ask yourself whether you really love it. There should be absolutely nothing in your life, right down to the bowl you eat your breakfast out of, that you don't absolutely adore. Use 'love' as the criterion to edit out everything that doesn't enhance, enrich, encourage or delight you.

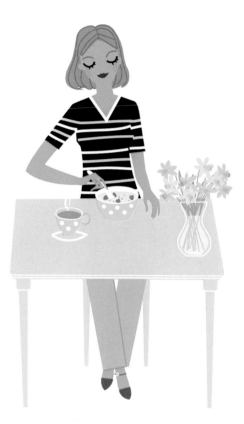

Act like a Girl Guide... and get into the habit of doing a daily good deed. It's far easier to believe you're a good person if you act like one, so start committing Random Acts of Kindness whenever you can. Make your day by making someone else's and record what you've done in your *Adore Yourself Slim* Travel Journal.

Get in the gratitude groove. As the Greek philosopher Epictetus once wrote: 'He is a wise man who does not grieve for the things which he has not, but rejoices for those which he has.' While you're brushing your teeth before bed, think of three things you're happy to be (such as funny, determined or enthusiastic), three things you've done well that day (not lost your temper with your kids, cooked a

healthy meal, smiled at a stranger) and three things you're grateful to have (your health, a loving partner, that bunch of daffodils). At the end of each week, write your favourites in your *Adore Yourself Slim* Travel Journal.

Fake it to make it. Think of the most confident and successful person you know and analyse how they dress, look and behave – and then start copying them. What you really feel inside doesn't count, because what you'll be telling the world is that you have unshakeable self-belief. And guess what? With nothing better to go on than what you tell them, other people will soon start treating you like a person who's confident and successful – which will boost your real confidence.

THE *ADORE YOURSELF SLIM* BODY MAP

Remember that song from the musical *Hair* called *I Got Life* that celebrated having every body part, from your arms right down to your liver? Well, we're going to employ the same tactics here to help you fall in love with your body as it is right here, right now. When you're slimming, it's all too easy to indulge in a bit of mental body-bashing and focus on the body parts you dislike, rather than making time to appreciate those you should be grateful for. So now I'd like you to use the Body Map outline, opposite, to analyse what you really love about your body. Colour in the hearts next to your favourite body parts – your glossy hair, your sparkling eyes, your megawatt smile, your shapely ankles – and fill in the explanations about why they're special to you.

This is an exercise in boosting your self-esteem and showing you that you already have lots to be thankful for. Whenever you feel discouraged, look at this Body Map and remind yourself of everything you *already* love about your body. Your mind is like a DVD player and you can choose which DVD to play. If you find yourself watching a DVD that depicts your frustration at still having less-than-lovely thighs, for example, use this Body Map to help you choose a different DVD in which you're spending time appreciating your slender calves or emerging hipbones. This thought-replacement technique is a great way to avoid the negative thinking that can so easily snowball into a comfort-eating fest.

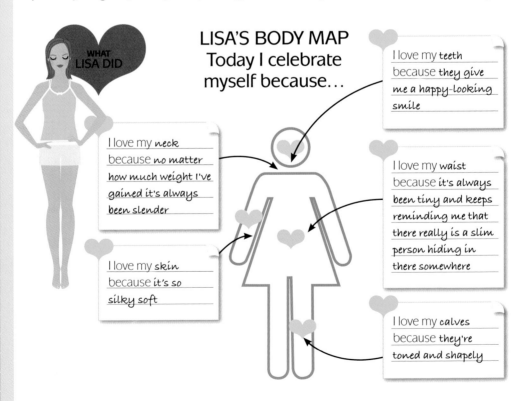

WHAT LISA DID

LISA'S BODY MAP
Today I celebrate myself because…

I love my teeth because they give me a happy-looking smile

I love my neck because no matter how much weight I've gained it's always been slender

I love my waist because it's always been tiny and keeps reminding me that there really is a slim person hiding in there somewhere

I love my skin because it's so silky soft

I love my calves because they're toned and shapely

YOUR BODY MAP
Today I celebrate myself because…

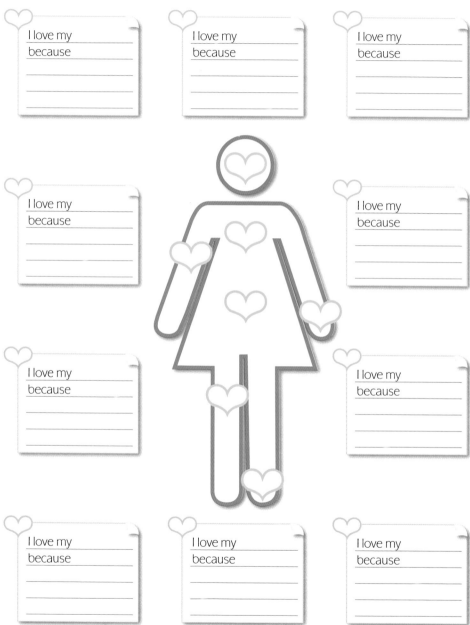

I love my
because

I love my
because

I love my
because

I love my
because

I love my
because

I love my
because

I love my
because

I love my
because

I love my
because

I love my
because

I love my
because

CREATE A GOAL GROUP

Losing weight can sometimes feel like a lonely journey: it can feel as if you're the only person in the entire world saying 'No' when the biscuits are being passed around or the dessert menu arrives. So a good tactic to ensure that your new weight-loss plan will be a success is to surround yourself with people who are backing your efforts 1,000% and who truly believe you'll achieve your goals. One way to do this is to put together a Goal Group of the people you can count on to motivate you – and who'll only be a phone call away if you need a bit of a pep talk. They can be anyone from an encouraging colleague (who'll raise an eyebrow if she spies you having a pastry for breakfast instead of muesli) to your best friend (who'll meet you for a run rather than a boozy night out) to a personal trainer (who'll make sure you do more sweating than chatting at the gym). Below is my own Goal Group and the reasons why I chose each member. Whenever I had a wobbly phase, it was comforting to look at this chart and know that I had a full team I could rely on to back me all the way.

WHAT LISA DID

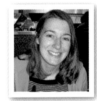

Graham Williams, my husband, because he encourages me to go running, praises me when I do and cooks me healthy food

Jenny Wood, my former colleague, because she nudged and nagged me into devising my weight-loss plan

Bridget Robinson, my slimming buddy (see page 38), because she's the world's most supportive friend and travels halfway around the globe to run marathons with me in fancy dress

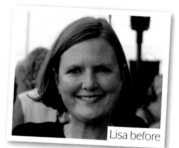

Lisa before

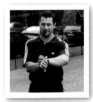

Coach Bronek, my fitness coach, because he's fanatical about exercise, fierce but funny and really believes that I can succeed at anything

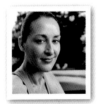

Sarah Maxwell, a celebrity personal trainer, because she's the only fitness professional I've ever met who understands that you can dislike working out just as much as you can't live without it

Kelly Beswick (left) and Tara Nathanson, my former colleagues, because they never ducked out of doing our lunchtime running sessions

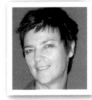

Lyndel Costain, my dietitian, because she helped me reach my goal of eating for wellbeing, not just weight loss

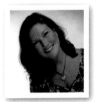

Jennie Francis, my former hypnotherapist, because she encouraged me to put myself first and permanently changed my relationship with food

MY GOAL GROUP

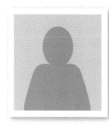

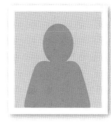

because
_____
_____
_____
Tel no _____

because
_____
_____
_____
Tel no _____

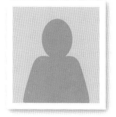

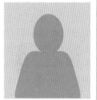

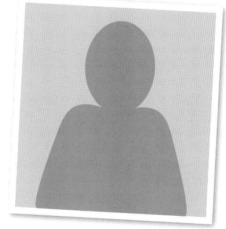

because
_____
_____
_____
Tel no _____

because
_____
_____
Tel no _____

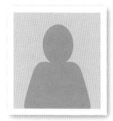

because
_____
_____
_____
Tel no _____

because
_____
_____
Tel no _____

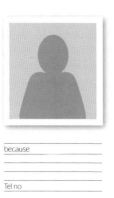

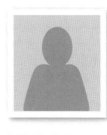

because
_____
_____
_____
Tel no _____

because
_____
_____
_____
Tel no _____

THE SLIMMING BUDDY'S STORY

'My name is Bridget Robinson and I'm Lisa's slimming buddy. The remarkable weight-loss journey we took together started a few years ago when, after a long period of steadily gaining weight, I overheard a friend's daughter, Laura, whom I hadn't seen for a year, saying to her mum: "Yes, I remember Bridg, but she's older and fatter than she was last year." It took a five-year-old's innocent remark to alert me to the fact that I needed to do something about being 2st 2lb (13.6kg) overweight. Of course, I was already aware that I had a problem (wearing elasticated skirts was a bit of a giveaway!), but awareness hadn't translated into action due to my ingenious rationalisations: I'd convinced myself that the project I was working on took precedence over healthy eating; that there was no time to exercise and that snacking wasn't only excusable but was actually required fuel for burning the midnight oil.

'Having identified the problem with Laura's help, I set about the next step of solving it by gathering all the information I could about healthy eating and exercise. Then, by a total coincidence, Lisa, a school friend who lives 4,000 miles away (I live in Canada, she lives in London), mentioned that she was embarking on a weight-loss plan, too, and suggested we become slimming buddies. I readily agreed and we began Skyping or emailing each other every fortnight. I regularly sent Lisa my Excel weight-loss graph and we traded slimming strategies. We also made sure our plan was liberally sprinkled with incentives to keep us motivated (I'll never forget Lisa sending me a fabulous mascara that served not only as a reward but as a reminder to always look my best). Our mega-reward for reaching Destination Dream Weight (as we called it) was a trip to Bordeaux, where we celebrated the culmination of our great, grand weight-loss adventure by running a festive fancy-dress marathon through the vineyards of Médoc, with me dressed as a ladybird and Lisa as a glorious butterfly.

MARATHON EFFORT

'My weight-loss journey was a lot like the marathon we ran – it's possible I could have done it alone, but it would have been a lot harder, a lot less joyful and no doubt would have taken a lot longer. It made all the difference having someone to encourage me through the challenging days, to celebrate the milestones and ultimately to cross the finish line with.' *Bridget Robinson*

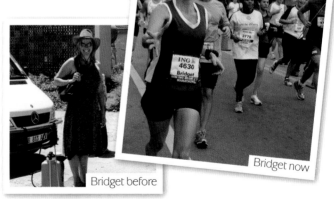

Bridget before

Bridget now

WHAT LISA'S HYPNOTHERAPY PATIENTS DID…

I run a care home and look after up to 14 residents with learning difficulties. I'm on call 24/7 and used comfort eating to de-stress. When I first saw Lisa, I'd pretty much given up hope of ever losing weight, but she encouraged me to put myself first for a change. Before, weight loss had always seemed like hard work, but Lisa made it sound exciting and I left my first hypnotherapy session thinking: 'Yeah, great, let's get it sorted!' I began to sit down whenever I ate, instead of eating on the hoof, and threw out the leftover party food from residents' birthdays instead of finishing it off. I also found time to exercise regularly and used my iPhone's calendar to remind myself to practise self-hypnosis and implement the three lifestyle changes I'd agreed to make during every hypnotherapy session. Losing over 3st (19kg) has boosted my confidence immeasurably and I now feel incredibly positive about the future.

Kirsty Brown, 42, care home manager, Croydon

Hypnotherapy literally changed my life. I was desperate when I came to see Lisa, as my job as a social worker was unbelievably stressful (in two years my caseload tripled!) and I felt I simply didn't have time to eat well or exercise. Lisa helped me realise that my 'poor me' thinking was holding me back, so I swapped it for a 'can-do' attitude and started doing things I loved, such as salsa dancing and tennis. I used all the techniques Lisa taught me, such as writing down my compliments, and set up a Goal Group of people who wanted me to succeed. One member was a stay-at-home mum whom I paid to cook me healthy meals, another was a colleague who'd answer my phone for me when I went out for my lunchtime walk. I also practised self-hypnosis every single day and enjoyed imagining the slim person I was slowly becoming, as Lisa suggested. I've lost 2st (12.7kg) overall so far and still have a way to go, but I'm already loving the new me.

Carmen Nel, 31, social worker, London

'HYPNOSIS HELPED ME LOSE 5ST/32KG'

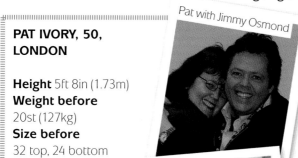

Pat with Jimmy Osmond

PAT IVORY, 50, LONDON

Height 5ft 8in (1.73m)
Weight before
20st (127kg)
Size before
32 top, 24 bottom
Weight now
15st (95.3kg)
Size now
18 top, 16 bottom
WEIGHT LOST
5st/32kg

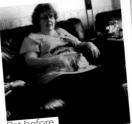

Pat before

'I've been an Osmonds fan since I was 12, when I fell in love with Donny. Chasing them all over the world has kept me young, but ironically it's also led me both to gain and lose a lot of weight. I was a normal weight at school, but when I left at 16 I exercised only occasionally and ate a lot of rubbish food, especially chocolate, and the pounds just kept creeping on. At 18 I went

to my first slimming club, and over the years I joined various different ones and kept going on fad diets. Each time I lost weight I'd later regain it – and more.

'In the 1980s and 1990s, I was lucky enough to get to know all of the Osmonds and became good friends with Jimmy. They made frequent appearances in the UK and I'd end up sitting in my car with my friends munching vast amounts of rubbish while we waited to see their shows. We used to joke that our motto was "Osmonds first, then food!" I gained about 2st (12.7kg) every decade until I was 20st (127kg). By the time I went to see Lisa, I was 49 and I'd decided that while I'd been fat at 20, 30 and 40, I didn't want to turn 50 and still be fat. I was also worried that I wouldn't be able to fit into the plane seat when I flew to Las Vegas to see The Osmonds.

SMALL CHANGES, BIG RESULTS

'Lisa didn't tell me to diet, she just encouraged me to commit to doing three things each session that would make me feel healthier. The first week I chose to start weaning myself off the diet cola I'd lived on for 30 years. I also decided to stop eating butter and have one portion of vegetables every day (at that time the only veggies I'd eat were tomatoes). No one was

Pat today

more surprised than I was when, after just one hypnotherapy session, I began eating vegetables and drinking several litres of water a day, having completely lost the taste for diet cola. I'd lost 4st (25.4kg) and regained it (and more) before, so I knew that this time I had to focus not just on what I ate but on changing my entire lifestyle and getting fitter. Which is why I decided to see a personal trainer, Shelley Baker, who encouraged me to go to the gym for 30 minutes five times a week and take up swimming. Being big, gyms and pools were two of my biggest fears, but I was so determined to succeed that I forced myself to go. I was actually on crutches at this point, having injured my foot, but I didn't let that hold me back. The first session nearly killed me, but I persevered because I knew Lisa and Shelley really cared about me succeeding. My husband Mick, friends and family were also all very supportive, though they didn't know what had happened to me and said they thought I'd been taken over by aliens! A month later, when I went to Vegas, I had no problem fitting into the plane seat, having lost over 1st (6.4kg).

ADDICTED TO EXERCISE

'As I continued to lose weight, everyday life became so much easier. It used to be incredibly difficult to go up stairs, but now I can easily do it. And whereas before I found it hard to bend over to do up my shoes, that's no longer a problem. But the greatest change has been in my attitude to exercise – I've discovered a whole new world of fun and challenging activities. I've recently completed a half-marathon bike ride and signed up to do a triathlon and two three-mile (5km) charity runs – and next year I've got my sights set on doing the New York City Marathon (I also want to take up surfing, try white-water rafting and learn to dance!). Later this year, when I hope to be 11st or 12st (70kg or 76.2kg), I'm going back to Vegas to see The Osmonds perform. I've had many photos taken with them over the years, but the only slim photo I have shows me with Donny when I was 18. I can't wait to be photographed with him again, as I'm sure he'll be really surprised at the new me!'

WHAT LISA THOUGHT

When I first met Pat she could barely walk, so I was impressed by her determination to change not only her eating habits but to take up exercise, too. Breaking down her ultimate goal of losing 9st (57.2kg) into three manageable tasks each session gave her the courage to tackle a weight problem that could easily have seemed overwhelming. I also gave Pat a copy of The Ten Slimming Commandments (see page 74), to give her new ideas for changing her lifestyle. What most impressed me about Pat was that after an initial rocky start when she told me she was continuing to eat chips because 'It's normal for me to do it', she embraced every challenge I set her and kept coming up with her own solutions to the obstacles she faced. One truly courageous thing she did was to allow her personal trainer Shelley to film her at her heaviest, so she'd remember how far she'd come when she got fitter. You can view footage of her remarkable transformation at http://fits-u-personaltraining.co.uk.

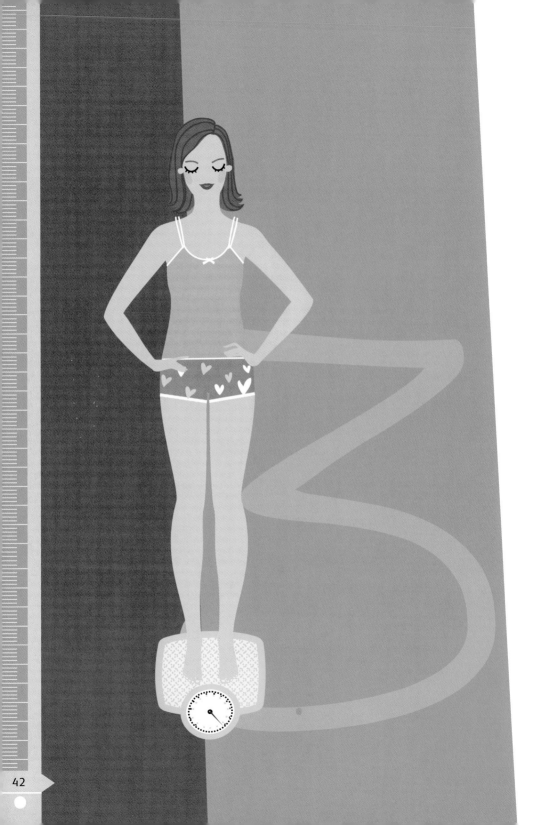

Chapter 3

SET YOUR
slimming
GOALS

This is a chapter that, like a beautiful city, you'll come back to time and time again. You'll use it to discover the real reasons why you've decided to slim and to set up a super-motivating reward system. You'll also write your weight and measurements in it regularly and experience the spine-tingling thrill of watching that line on your Weight-Loss Graph dip ever lower. And when you finally reach Destination Dream Weight and are doing all the things you dreamt of doing (which you'll have recorded on your Want-To-Do List), it'll be the logbook you look back on with great pride to remind you of the route you took to get there…

THE 'WHAT DO I *REALLY* WANT?' SELF-HYPNOSIS SESSION

I've already mentioned my all-time favourite quote: 'Goals are dreams with deadlines', so in this chapter you're going to access your innermost dreams and desires by doing some self-hypnosis before you set yourself some deadlines to help make your dreams a reality. You've already experienced what it's like to be hypnotised when you listened to Track 1 on the CD, but now I'm going to teach you how to hypnotise yourself, without my help.

1 **Find a quiet place where you're unlikely to be disturbed** and make yourself comfortable.

2 **Close your eyes and then start counting down from ten to one,** silently saying each number as you breathe out. With each exhalation, allow any unnecessary nervous tension to flow out of your body, like the sand in an egg-timer. Don't worry if you don't feel as deeply relaxed as you did when you listened to the CD – it's not uncommon to find it harder to go into a self-induced hypnotic state than if you're hypnotised by a hypnotherapist.

3 **Now imagine yourself in your Favourite Place of Relaxation** (a real or imaginary place where you feel completely relaxed, safe and secure). Hear the sounds, smell the fragrances, touch your surroundings and re-create that wonderfully relaxed feeling you had when you were last there (or imagine how you'd feel if you were blissfully relaxed). Spend as long as you like enjoying this feeling of profound relaxation. If other thoughts start to distract you, simply acknowledge them before returning your focus to your Favourite Place of Relaxation.

4 **Remaining completely relaxed, I'd like you now to focus your attention on the reasons that you want to lose weight.** Think about how you'll feel when you're slimmer, what you'll look like, what outfits you'll wear, the activities you'll be participating in, what you'll be able to do then that you may not be able to do now. Then start to draw up a list in your mind of the short-term, medium-term and lifelong reasons why you'd like to be slimmer and healthier.

5 **To awaken from the session, start counting from one to ten,** silently saying each number on every inhalation. Open your eyes when your reach ten and have a lovely long stretch.

6 **Now you're ready to fill in the chart opposite.** If you get stuck, read through the reasons I came up with in my own What Do I *Really* Want? session overleaf for some inspiration…

MY REASONS TO BE SLIM

SHORT-TERM REASONS	TIME FRAME

MEDIUM-TERM REASONS	TIME FRAME

LIFELONG REASONS	TIME FRAME

LISA'S REASONS TO BE SLIM

SHORT-TERM REASONS	TIME FRAME
1 To enjoy being complimented	Immediately
2 To surprise my husband Graham when he returns midway through his three-month posting in Bangladesh	6 weeks
3 To buy gorgeous new clothes for summer	8 weeks
4 To get my cheekbones, hipbones and collarbones back	4 weeks
5 To feel more comfortable in my clothes	2 weeks
6 To regain control of what I'm eating	Immediately
7 To be happy being photographed	4 weeks

MEDIUM-TERM REASONS	TIME FRAME
1 To earn even more compliments	11st 11lb (75kg)
2 To be able to buy my first pair of jeans in 27 years!	11st 5lb (72kg)
3 To be able to run a marathon in under five hours	TBC
4 To look better at 40 than I did at 25!	25 weeks
5 To celebrate reaching Destination Dream Weight with my slimming buddy Bridget in Prague	10st 8lb (66kg)
6 To finally reach my goal and know I only have to worry about losing a pound or two if I gain weight, rather than tens of pounds	10st 8lb (66kg)

LIFELONG REASONS

1 To always be able to buy the clothes I like rather than the ones that are able to offer the best camouflage

2 To find that everything's easier when you're slimmer, from shopping to sightseeing to walking up stairs

3 To be lighter on my feet when running and so avoid injury

4 To enjoy 50 years of good health by not getting diabetes, heart disease and cancer, or having a stroke

5 To be fabulous at 50, 60, 70, 80 and 99! And always to look, act and feel younger than my biological age

CHOOSE YOUR REWARDS

Now that you know why you *really* want to be slim, it's time to choose the rewards that will help to spur you on to achieving your goals. To keep myself motivated when I started the programme, I decided to give myself the most invigorating, uplifting start to every day by using a grapefruit body scrub in the shower. I also started going to bed 30 minutes earlier each night. And a few times a week, I used a self-tan body moisturiser to give my skin a sun-kissed glow. These mini-treats gave me the 'I'm worth it' feel-good factor that helped to keep me on track when the going got tough.

TANGIBLE TREATS

Besides the daily rewards, I also spent a good hour or two constructing a list of rewards for achieving different weight-loss goals. There were rewards for dropping a dress size (a luxury mascara and a pretty new top), rewards for moving from one category on the BMI (body mass index) chart to the next (a gorgeous new dress) and for significant weight-loss milestones, such as losing a stone or 10kg (I used both imperial and metric milestones as an excuse to fit in a few extra rewards!). I found the most effective rewards were the tangible ones, such as buying a new item of clothing, as they not only served as a permanent

souvenir of hitting a target but also got me lots of compliments that I could add to my collection (see page 146), and acted as an incentive to inspire me to keep the weight off permanently.

Now it's time for you to set up your own reward system – choose from the options below (or dream up your own) and then write your choices on the chart overleaf.

DAILY TREATS FOR STICKING TO THE PROGRAMME

▉ Use an invigorating body scrub and loofah in the bath or shower.
▉ Spend ten minutes in your garden or a park connecting with nature.
▉ Read a chapter of the latest page-turner.
▉ Apply a self-tan body moisturiser.
▉ Sit in a public place and enjoy watching the world go by.

WEIGHT-LOSS REWARDS

▉ Have a blissful massage, facial or manicure.
▉ Get that lipstick/eyeshadow/perfume/earrings/necklace you've had your eye on.
▉ Visit a comedy club with a group of friends and laugh till you're breathless.
▉ Sign up for a course: scuba diving, wine tasting, yoga, rock climbing, Indian head massage, orienteering, art history.
▉ Shop for a new outfit – and enjoy choosing it in a smaller size.
▉ Buy yourself the latest must-have CD/DVD/novel.
▉ Subscribe to an inspiring health or fitness magazine.
▉ Treat yourself to an adventurous new haircut.
▉ Book yourself a romantic weekend break or exotic holiday.

YOUR WEIGHT-LOSS REWARD SCHEDULE

Getting to	kg/	st	lb	
Reward				Date achieved

Getting to	kg/	st	lb	
Reward				Date achieved

Getting to	kg/	st	lb	
Reward				Date achieved

Getting out of the Very Overweight/Obese zone on the BMI chart (see page 50)

Reward	Date achieved

Getting out of the Overweight zone on the BMI chart (see page 50)

Reward	Date achieved

Getting to my 5% weight-loss target of	kg/	st	lb
Reward		Date achieved	

Getting to my 10% weight-loss target of	kg/	st	lb
Reward		Date achieved	

Dropping a dress size (size	to	)
Reward	Date achieved	

Dropping a dress size (size	to	)
Reward	Date achieved	

Dropping a dress size (size	to	)
Reward	Date achieved	

Losing my first	inches/	centimetres
Reward	Date achieved	

Losing	inches/	centimetres
Reward	Date achieved	

Losing	inches/	centimetres
Reward	Date achieved	

Sticking to the changes I've chosen on my Adoption Certificate (see page 83)

Reward	Date achieved

Sticking to the additional changes I've chosen on my Adoption Certificate (see page 83)

Reward	Date achieved

GETTING TO MY GOAL WEIGHT OF	**KG/**	**ST**	**LB**	**CM/INCH-LOSS TARGET**
MEGA-REWARD				**DATE ACHIEVED**

MADE TO MEASURE

Now it's time to take stock of where you're at right now so that you can measure your progress as you follow the *Adore Yourself Slim* plan. I've included space to record not only your BMI (body mass index) and weight but your measurements, too. BMI has received a bad press in recent years, as very muscular people such as athletes are sometimes classified as obese since they're so heavy in proportion to their height. However, for most of us (except the very frail or muscle-bound) it's a really useful tool to give us at least a ballpark figure of what we should be aiming for.

WEIGHT AND BMI (BODY MASS INDEX)

■ Measure your height and your weight while naked and then fill in these figures on page 51, along with your current dress size, the date and your weigh-in time (aim for the same time each day). Now look at the Body Mass Index Chart, overleaf, to determine your BMI and healthy weight range and then fill that in, too, along with your 5% and 10% weight-loss goals, your Destination Dream Weight (ultimate *realistic* target weight) and your desired BMI and dress size.
■ A healthy weight range is a BMI of 18.5–24.9. If your BMI is between 25 and 29.9, you're overweight. If it's 30 or more, you're very overweight (medically called 'obese') and losing some weight will benefit your health. It's a good idea to visit your GP for a health check (he or she can also offer extra support if you need it). Some people find weight management harder than others.
■ For a really inspirational, graphic picture of your weight-loss progress, fill in the results on the graph on page 52 and keep updating it every week.

▶ **10% = SUCCESS!**
Losing weight has enormous health benefits and the best news of all is that you don't have to be thin, your ideal weight or even within your healthy weight range to benefit from significant health improvements. Reducing your bodyweight by just 5% to 10% can make a big difference: if someone who weighs 100kg (15st 10lb), for example, loses 10% of their bodyweight (10kg/1st 8lb), they can expect to *halve*[1] their risk of developing diabetes plus a 40% reduction in their risk of dying from an obesity-related cancer. It would also benefit a whole range of health problems, from polycystic ovarian syndrome to back pain to high blood pressure to snoring!

■ Finally, turn to page 148 at the back of this book and fill in the relevant details on Day 1 of your *Adore Yourself Slim* Travel Journal.
■ Experts are divided about how often you should weigh yourself. I simply loved doing it every day and shot out of bed to discover what progress I'd made. But if you're the kind of person who takes it to heart if there's no change in your weight (which may simply be due to something like where you are in your menstrual cycle), it's probably best to only do so once a week, as that way your weight loss will have had a chance to accumulate.

BODY MASS INDEX CHART

BMI	UNDERWEIGHT				HEALTHY WEIGHT RANGE						OVERWEIGHT					VERY OVERWEIGHT/OBESE					
	15	16	17	18	19	20	21	22	23	24	25	26	27	28	29	30	31	32	33	34	35
4ft 10in 1.47m	5st 1lb 32kg	5st 5lb 35kg	5st 12lb 37kg	6st 2lb 39kg	6st 6lb 41kg	6st 11lb 43kg	7st 1lb 45kg	7st 8lb 48kg	7st 12lb 50kg	8st 3lb 52kg	8st 7lb 54kg	8st 11lb 56kg	9st 2lb 58kg	9st 8lb 61kg	9st 13lb 63kg	10st 3lb 65kg	10st 8lb 67kg	10st 12lb 69kg	11st 3lb 71kg	11st 7lb 73kg	12st 76kg
4ft 11in 1.50m	5st 5lb 34kg	5st 9lb 36kg	6st 38kg	6st 6lb 41kg	6st 11lb 43kg	7st 1lb 45kg	7st 6lb 47kg	7st 12lb 50kg	8st 3lb 52kg	8st 7lb 54kg	8st 11lb 56kg	9st 4lb 59kg	9st 8lb 61kg	9st 13lb 63kg	10st 3lb 65kg	10st 10lb 68kg	11st 70kg	11st 5lb 72kg	11st 9lb 74kg	12st 2lb 77kg	12st 6lb 79kg
5ft 1.52m	5st 7lb 35kg	5st 12lb 37kg	6st 2lb 39kg	6st 9lb 42kg	6st 13lb 44kg	7st 3lb 46kg	7st 10lb 49kg	8st 51kg	8st 5lb 53kg	8st 9lb 55kg	9st 2lb 58kg	9st 6lb 60kg	9st 11lb 62kg	10st 3lb 65kg	10st 8lb 67kg	10st 12lb 69kg	11st 5lb 72kg	11st 9lb 74kg	12st 76kg	12st 6lb 79kg	12st 11lb 81kg
5ft 1in 1.55m	5st 9lb 36kg	6st 38kg	6st 6lb 41kg	6st 11lb 43kg	7st 3lb 46kg	7st 8lb 48kg	7st 12lb 50kg	8st 5lb 53kg	8st 9lb 55kg	9st 2lb 58kg	9st 6lb 60kg	9st 11lb 62kg	10st 3lb 65kg	10st 8lb 67kg	11st 70kg	11st 5lb 72kg	11st 9lb 74kg	12st 2lb 77kg	12st 6lb 79kg	12st 13lb 82kg	13st 3lb 84kg
5ft 2in 1.57m	5st 12lb 37kg	6st 2lb 39kg	6st 9lb 42kg	6st 13lb 44kg	7st 6lb 47kg	7st 10lb 49kg	8st 3lb 52kg	8st 7lb 54kg	9st 57kg	9st 4lb 59kg	9st 11lb 62kg	10st 1lb 64kg	10st 8lb 67kg	10st 12lb 69kg	11st 3lb 71kg	11st 9lb 74kg	12st 76kg	12st 6lb 79kg	12st 11lb 81kg	13st 3lb 84kg	13st 8lb 86kg
5ft 3in 1.6m	6st 38kg	6st 6lb 41kg	6st 13lb 44kg	7st 3lb 46kg	7st 10lb 49kg	8st 51kg	8st 7lb 54kg	8st 11lb 56kg	9st 4lb 59kg	9st 8lb 61kg	10st 1lb 64kg	10st 8lb 67kg	10st 12lb 69kg	11st 5lb 72kg	11st 9lb 74kg	12st 2lb 77kg	12st 6lb 79kg	12st 13lb 82kg	13st 3lb 84kg	13st 10lb 87kg	14st 2lb 90kg
5ft 4in 1.63m	6st 4lb 40kg	6st 9lb 42kg	7st 1lb 45kg	7st 8lb 48kg	7st 12lb 50kg	8st 5lb 53kg	8st 11lb 56kg	9st 2lb 58kg	9st 8lb 61kg	10st 1lb 64kg	10st 6lb 66kg	10st 12lb 69kg	11st 5lb 72kg	11st 9lb 74kg	12st 2lb 77kg	12st 8lb 80kg	12st 13lb 82kg	13st 5lb 85kg	13st 12lb 88kg	14st 2lb 90kg	14st 9lb 93kg
5ft 5in 1.65m	6st 6lb 41kg	6st 13lb 44kg	7st 3lb 46kg	7st 10lb 49kg	8st 3lb 52kg	8st 7lb 54kg	9st 57kg	9st 6lb 60kg	9st 13lb 63kg	10st 3lb 65kg	10st 10lb 68kg	11st 3lb 71kg	11st 9lb 74kg	12st 76kg	12st 6lb 79kg	12st 13lb 82kg	13st 3lb 84kg	13st 10lb 87kg	14st 2lb 90kg	14st 9lb 93kg	14st 13lb 95kg
5ft 6in 1.68m	6st 9lb 42kg	7st 1lb 45kg	7st 8lb 48kg	8st 51kg	8st 7lb 54kg	8st 11lb 56kg	9st 4lb 59kg	9st 11lb 62kg	10st 3lb 65kg	10st 10lb 68kg	11st 3lb 71kg	11st 7lb 73kg	12st 76kg	12st 6lb 79kg	12st 13lb 82kg	13st 5lb 85kg	13st 10lb 87kg	14st 2lb 90kg	14st 9lb 93kg	15st 2lb 96kg	15st 8lb 99kg
5ft 7in 1.7m	6st 11lb 43kg	7st 3lb 46kg	7st 10lb 49kg	8st 3lb 52kg	8st 9lb 55kg	9st 2lb 58kg	9st 8lb 61kg	10st 1lb 64kg	10st 6lb 66kg	10st 12lb 69kg	11st 5lb 72kg	11st 11lb 75kg	12st 4lb 78kg	12st 11lb 81kg	13st 3lb 84kg	13st 10lb 87kg	14st 2lb 90kg	14st 7lb 92kg	14st 13lb 95kg	15st 6lb 98kg	15st 13lb 101kg
5ft 8in 1.73m	7st 1lb 45kg	7st 8lb 48kg	8st 51kg	8st 7lb 54kg	9st 57kg	9st 6lb 60kg	9st 13lb 63kg	10st 6lb 66kg	10st 12lb 69kg	11st 5lb 72kg	11st 11lb 75kg	12st 4lb 78kg	12st 11lb 81kg	13st 3lb 84kg	13st 10lb 87kg	14st 2lb 90kg	14st 9lb 93kg	15st 2lb 96kg	15st 8lb 99kg	16st 1lb 102kg	16st 7lb 105kg
5ft 9in 1.75m	7st 3lb 46kg	7st 10lb 49kg	8st 3lb 52kg	8st 9lb 55kg	9st 2lb 58kg	9st 8lb 61kg	10st 1lb 64kg	10st 8lb 67kg	11st 70kg	11st 9lb 74kg	12st 2lb 77kg	12st 8lb 80kg	13st 1lb 83kg	13st 8lb 86kg	14st 89kg	14st 7lb 92kg	14st 13lb 95kg	15st 6lb 98kg	15st 13lb 101kg	16st 5lb 104kg	16st 12lb 107kg
5ft 10in 1.78m	7st 8lb 48kg	8st 51kg	8st 7lb 54kg	9st 57kg	9st 6lb 60kg	9st 13lb 63kg	10st 8lb 67kg	11st 70kg	11st 7lb 73kg	12st 76kg	12st 6lb 79kg	12st 13lb 82kg	13st 8lb 86kg	14st 89kg	14st 7lb 92kg	14st 13lb 95kg	15st 6lb 98kg	15st 13lb 101kg	16st 7lb 105kg	17st 108kg	17st 7lb 111kg
5ft 11in 1.8m	7st 10lb 49kg	8st 3lb 52kg	8st 9lb 55kg	9st 2lb 58kg	9st 11lb 62kg	10st 3lb 65kg	10st 10lb 68kg	11st 3lb 71kg	11st 11lb 75kg	12st 4lb 78kg	12st 11lb 81kg	13st 3lb 84kg	13st 12lb 88kg	14st 5lb 91kg	14st 11lb 94kg	15st 4lb 97kg	15st 10lb 100kg	16st 5lb 104kg	16st 12lb 107kg	17st 5lb 110kg	17st 11lb 113kg
6ft 1.83m	7st 12lb 50kg	8st 7lb 54kg	9st 57kg	9st 6lb 60kg	10st 1lb 64kg	10st 8lb 67kg	11st 70kg	11st 9lb 74kg	12st 2lb 77kg	12st 8lb 80kg	13st 3lb 84kg	13st 10lb 87kg	14st 2lb 90kg	14st 11lb 94kg	15st 4lb 97kg	15st 10lb 100kg	16st 5lb 104kg	16st 12lb 107kg	17st 7lb 111kg	17st 13lb 114kg	18st 6lb 117kg

MY WEIGHT AND BMI

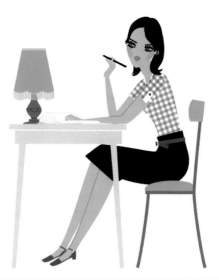

My height _____

My healthy weight range _____

My 5% weight-loss target _____

My 10% weight-loss target _____

Destination Dream Weight _____

My desired BMI _____

My desired dress size _____

	DATE AND WEIGH-IN TIME	WEIGHT	WEIGHT LOSS	BMI	DRESS SIZE
Today			0		
After 1 week					
After 2 weeks					
After 3 weeks					
After 4 weeks					
After 5 weeks					
After 6 weeks					
After 7 weeks					
After 8 weeks					
After 9 weeks					
After 10 weeks					
After 3 months					
After 4 months					
After 5 months					
After 6 months					
After 9 months					
After a year					
After 18 months					
After 2 years					

MY WEIGHT-LOSS GRAPH Each block = 1kg or 2lb

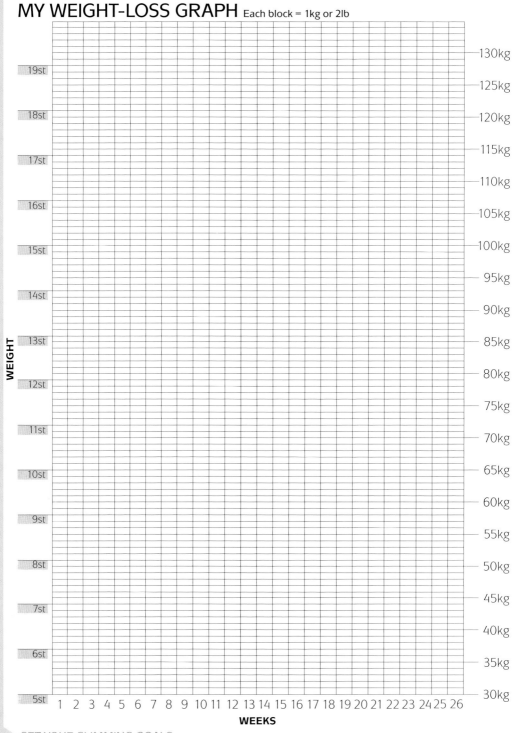

WEIGHT

19st — 130kg
— 125kg
18st — 120kg
— 115kg
17st — 110kg
16st — 105kg
15st — 100kg
— 95kg
14st — 90kg
13st — 85kg
— 80kg
12st — 75kg
11st — 70kg
— 65kg
10st — 60kg
9st — 55kg
8st — 50kg
— 45kg
7st — 40kg
6st — 35kg
5st — 30kg

1 2 3 4 5 6 7 8 9 10 11 12 13 14 15 16 17 18 19 20 21 22 23 24 25 26
WEEKS

SET YOUR SLIMMING GOALS

MY MEASUREMENTS

	DATE	CHEST	WAIST	HIPS	THIGH	ARM
Today						
After 1 week						
After 2 weeks						
After 3 weeks						
After 4 weeks						
After 5 weeks						
After 6 weeks						
After 7 weeks						
After 8 weeks						
After 9 weeks						
After 10 weeks						
After 3 months						
After 4 months						
After 5 months						
After 6 months						
After 9 months						
After a year						
After 18 months						
After 2 years						

HOW TO TAKE YOUR MEASUREMENTS

Use a tape measure to take accurate measurements of your chest, waist, hips, thigh and upper arm – it's important to take readings from exactly the same place each time – and then fill them in on the chart above.

WHAT MEASUREMENTS MEAN

Not only is measuring your body a very motivating way to see how you're slimming down and toning up but knowing your waist measurement is also a very important way to assess your health, because carrying excess weight around your stomach (often called being 'apple-shaped') is linked to an increased risk of type-2 diabetes, high blood pressure and raised cholesterol.

Ideally, women should aim for a waist measurement of under 81cm/32in, whereas for men it's 94cm/37in. A waist measurement of 81–88cm/32–35in in women (94-102cm/37-40in for men) carries an increased risk to health; and more than 88cm/35in (more than 102cm/40in for men) carries a greatly increased risk to health.

YOUR WANT-TO-DO LIST

We're all too familiar with 'to-do' lists – I'm a big fan (you'll have noticed that this book is full of them), but often they can take over your life and result in you not doing the things you really love in favour of the things you feel you ought/should/must do. When you're overweight, it's tempting to postpone doing lots of things as you promise yourself that one day, when you're slimmer, everything from meeting your soulmate to getting that promotion to taking up the tango will be easier. I call this the 'I'll do it when I'm slim syndrome' and if you're not careful it can put happiness on hold indefinitely (if I'd waited until I was my dream weight I'd have missed out on running eight marathons while I was overweight, and marathon running is one of the things that has given me the most joy over the past 12 years). This attitude can be a symptom of low self-esteem or an excuse not to do things (a way of stopping you feeling that you've failed because you haven't even tried). So we're going to cure you of it right now. Just because you're overweight at the moment doesn't mean that you can't start living life to the full right this very second.

In the space provided opposite, I'd now like you to create your own Want-To-Do List by writing down every fun, silly, glorious, crazy-sounding dream or ambition you've ever had (such as learning to Rollerblade, wearing a bikini again, going on a hot date, discovering how to cook amazing meals, running a three-mile/5km fun run or climbing Mount Kilimanjaro) and setting yourself a date by which you'll have achieved it. And remember, don't put off doing any of this a moment longer (or feel guilty about allowing yourself to indulge in the things that give you pleasure) – being happier on a day-to-day basis is key to staying positive during your weight-loss journey and will help those pounds melt away. In addition, every time you do something that challenges (or scares!) you, you're expanding your comfort zone, which will give you the courage to tackle bigger challenges – and additional confidence in your ability to make the changes that will allow you to lose weight.

I DREAM OF...	... BY THIS DATE	DATE ACHIEVED

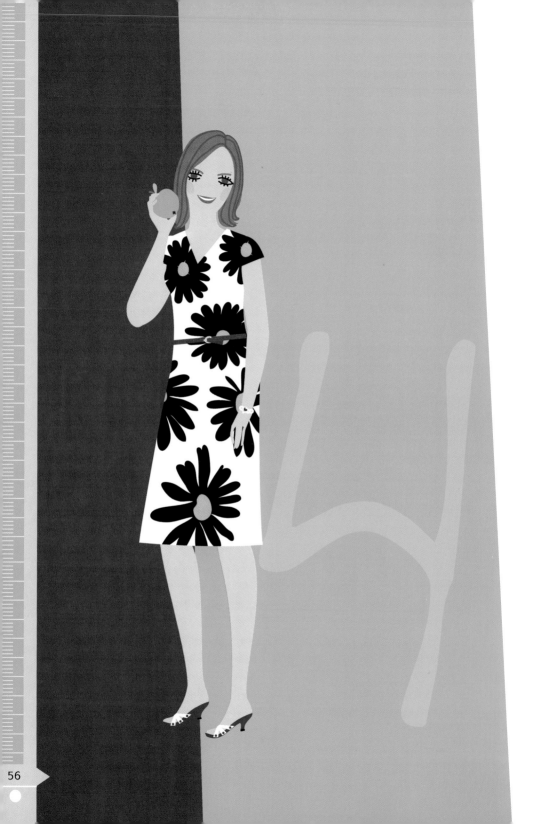

Chapter 4

EATyourself SLIM

Now for more detail about the yummy, can't-live-without, but tricky-to-manage-because-it's-everywhere part of our lives – food! In this chapter I'll introduce you to the *Adore Yourself Slim* Eating Plan, a moderate-carb plan devised by leading dietitian Lyndel Costain that's so simple you can memorise it in minutes. Not only will it help you lose weight but you'll feel more energetic than you've done for ages! There's also a shopping list to make it easy to buy healthy groceries, plus loads of information on how to handle those pesky hunger pangs. This chapter also includes some of the most mouthwatering recipes you'll ever come across – be prepared to forget dreary diet food for ever and delight in delicious, nutritious food again...

HOW THE *ADORE YOURSELF SLIM* EATING PLAN WAS BORN

Ever feel bombarded by often-conflicting nutrition advice that makes embracing a healthy diet feel really daunting and overwhelming? And frustrated when you think you're doing the right thing but the weight just still won't budge? I know how you're feeling because, as I found out, that tuna mayo baguette I'd been having for lunch in a misguided attempt to be 'good' turned out to contain the same number of calories as a kebab! Yes, really!

By the time I embarked on my healthy-eating plan I felt hopeless, having failed so many times before that I didn't know where to start. As I mentioned previously, my turning point came when I used Phase 1 of a low-carb diet as a basis for my new eating habits. However, I wasn't keen on the way it encouraged the use of sugar substitutes and featured too many time-consuming recipes, so I eliminated sweeteners and cooked simple, non-recipe food instead. My mum had been advised to change her eating habits radically when she'd been diagnosed with breast cancer, so I decided to adopt her suggestions, too, and chose to eat the most colourful array of vegetables possible, while generally avoiding anything containing additives or preservatives. And so,

through trial and error, I came up with an easy-to-remember, guilt-free eating plan that ticked most of the nutritional boxes. That plan helped me to lose just over 2½st (16.3kg) in just two-and-a-half months without ever feeling hungry (and unlike the occasions when I'd slimmed before, I could sense my body was loving what I was doing).

EAT FOR HEALTH, NOT JUST WEIGHT LOSS

And then, as I mentioned before in the introduction, I regained all the weight I'd lost, plus 4lb (2kg) more, while studying for my two hypnotherapy diplomas.

So by the time I was ready to tackle my weight problem once and for all, I felt I knew everything I needed to do to lose weight successfully. Except there was one thing missing: I wasn't sure my eating plan was 100% healthy. Was it a problem, I wondered, that I never ate fruit, for example? (The low-carb diet cut out fruit for only the first two weeks, but I hadn't got around to reintroducing it.) And was I depriving myself of vital nutrients by failing to eat potatoes, rice, pasta and bread? My mother's successful battle against cancer had taught me that nothing's more important than your health, and this time I wasn't prepared to compromise on my nutrition simply to be slim. I also wanted this to be the last time I ever lost a large amount of weight, so I was determined to follow an eating plan that was healthy enough to stick to for life. So I turned to Lyndel Costain, whose magazine articles I'd edited for years. One of the best-known registered dietitians in the UK, she has over 20 years' experience working in the National Health Service and as a nutrition consultant. Lyndel also advises and trains other health professionals in the field of weight management, has written five books and has made numerous TV and radio appearances, so I knew I was in safe hands.

'When Lisa asked me to check that her eating plan was as sensible as she hoped it was, I fine-tuned it to make it even more nutritious and balanced,' says Lyndel. 'I liked her "eat for health, not just weight loss" approach, but encouraged her to include more nutritious carbohydrates (at least three portions a day) and to reintroduce fruit. Like Lisa's original plan, my plan is

> 66 I wanted this to be the last time I ever lost a large amount of weight, so I was determined to follow an eating plan that was healthy enough to stick to for life 99

high in filling vegetables, but it's *moderate* (not low) in carbs. Lisa was adamant that cutting back on carbs had been key to her success, so I found a way for her to have a plan that limited carbs, but not so strictly. I felt this was essential because nutritious carbohydrates not only fuel exercise but contain fibre, B vitamins, minerals and beneficial antioxidants, which research[1] shows work together to offer heart, weight, blood sugar and digestive health benefits.'

While this plan certainly worked for me, helping me to lose 3½st (22kg), Lyndel and I aren't saying it's the single best way to eat to lose weight. What does seem to work best, though, according to Lyndel, is an overall approach that helps you build the skills to make healthy changes that are sustainable for you in the long term. We're all different, and you may well decide to follow another healthy weight-loss plan that you think will work for you (or even attend a slimming group), while using the other motivational strategies, hypnosis tracks and exercise routines in this book. So don't feel you have to follow this plan rigidly – simply use it as a guide to develop your own healthy-eating plan tailored around the healthy foods you love.

AN EVIDENCE-BASED APPROACH

'While health-promoting weight loss and maintenance is possible using a high-carbohydrate, moderate-protein, low-fat approach,' says Lyndel, 'an increasing body of research is also pointing towards the merits of using the moderate-carb, higher-protein, low-fat approach that Lisa adopted. For example, the early results of a large Europe-wide weight-loss study[2] found that a higher-protein, low-fat dietary approach was the most successful way to help maintain weight loss. What's more, an Australian study[3] has found that a higher protein intake was linked to better weight-loss maintenance over 12 months.'

If you have a medical problem, take medication, are under 18 or are pregnant or breastfeeding, please seek health-professional or medical advice before making changes to your diet or exercise patterns. Pregnancy is not a time to lose weight. The eating plans in this book are guidelines only and are not intended as individualised nutritional advice. Discuss any specific health, weight or dietary concerns with your doctor or dietitian.

WHAT'S SO SPECIAL ABOUT THE *ADORE YOURSELF SLIM* EATING PLAN?

YOU'LL LOSE WEIGHT SLOWLY – BUT PERMANENTLY

The *Adore Yourself Slim* Eating Plan will help most women slim at a healthy rate of about 1–2lb (0.5–1kg) a week, though you may lose a bit more in the first couple of weeks, mainly due to additional fluid loss. Losing weight slowly is the best way to ensure that new healthy habits become entrenched and the weight stays off.

YOU'LL BE FOLLOWING A PROVEN PLAN DESIGNED BY A TOP DIETITIAN

This eating plan is about enjoying more of the foods that protect and nourish your body (and mind), regulate your appetite and metabolism, and promote good health. It includes all the great stuff like antioxidants, your five-a-day of fruit and veg, calcium, vitamins, nutritious carbohydrates, healthy fats, protein and fibre – and at the same time it's calorie-controlled, as there is no special magic to weight loss, despite what some 'diets' might tell you. You'll notice that, unlike some eating plans, no food groups are eliminated entirely – that's because there is no scientific basis for doing so, as all food groups contain nutrients that are essential for optimum health. Reading about the science behind an eating strategy can be confusing (and boring!), so I asked Lyndel to ensure that the plan offered good nutrition and state-of-the-art expertise, but not to go into too much detail as to how it worked. But rest assured, there's evidence-based research to back up all of Lyndel's recommendations (see page 172). Our overall approach also meets best-practice guidance for weight-management programmes as recommended by the UK National Institute for Health and Clinical Excellence (NICE)[4].

YOU'LL NEVER BE HUNGRY

'We eat for many different reasons, but people often say that hunger is a key factor when they find it hard to manage their weight,' says Lyndel. 'Foods that help us feel fuller for longer (such as meals and snacks that are a good source of protein and fibre, along with some nutritious carbohydrates, to give slow, steady rises and falls in our blood sugar) can make a real difference when we want to be more in control around the convenient and comforting food we're so often surrounded by.'
This plan is full of these foods and food combinations, to help your body – and mind – better manage hunger.

YOU'LL EAT MINDFULLY

This plan aims to turn every meal into a body-nurturing ritual by encouraging you to:
- keep to a regular daily meal routine, starting with breakfast (eating breakfast is one of the main healthy habits research[5] consistently links to keeping weight off, thanks to its appetite-regulating benefits).
- eat at roughly the same times each day.
- aim for three meals and two snacks daily.
- never go for more than four or five hours without a meal or snack.
- sit down to eat, ideally at a table, and avoid distractions (turn off the TV, put away the paper, close your laptop – according to one study[6], people eat up to 44% more when they're glued to the television, and the more entertaining the programme, the more they eat, as they're too distracted to notice how much they've eaten).
- take small bites, eat slowly, chew well and really savour your food. This will give your internal appetite regulators time to kick in and tell your brain to stop eating[7].
- eat with others whenever you can – food also nourishes the soul.

YOU'LL ENJOY TREATS

This plan includes a variety of foods from the main food groups plus small amounts of 'treat' foods, such as wine or chocolate (hurrah!), as research[8] suggests that flexible rather than rigid eating plans work best and help you maintain a healthy relationship with food. This is known as *'flexible restraint'* and is key to this programme. It means making healthy choices most of the time, but building in some favourite foods, guilt-free, as no foods are forbidden. This helps manage any feelings of deprivation, and 'What the heck' thinking ('I've been "naughty" so I may as well keep eating'!). We suggest you choose the vast

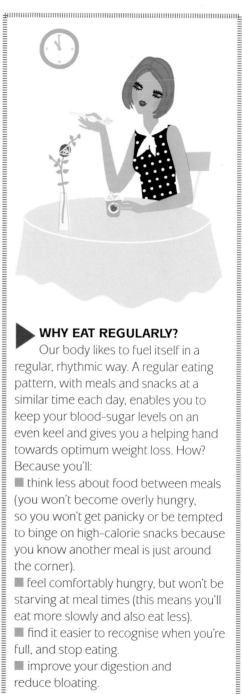

▶ WHY EAT REGULARLY?

Our body likes to fuel itself in a regular, rhythmic way. A regular eating pattern, with meals and snacks at a similar time each day, enables you to keep your blood-sugar levels on an even keel and gives you a helping hand towards optimum weight loss. How? Because you'll:
- think less about food between meals (you won't become overly hungry, so you won't get panicky or be tempted to binge on high-calorie snacks because you know another meal is just around the corner).
- feel comfortably hungry, but won't be starving at meal times (this means you'll eat more slowly and also eat less).
- find it easier to recognise when you're full, and stop eating.
- improve your digestion and reduce bloating.

majority of the foods you eat from those listed, as they're nutrient dense and good for helping to regulate your appetite and keep calories in check. While I was actively losing weight, I chose to stay right off alcohol as it dissolved my best-laid plans (willpower is soluble in alcohol!) and added calories I didn't want. You may choose that approach, too, though the plan allows for a small amount daily.

YOU'LL HAVE AT LEAST FIVE PORTIONS OF FRUIT AND VEG DAILY

YOU'LL EAT PROTEIN AT EVERY MEAL

Protein is one of the slimmer's best friends, as it helps us to feel fuller for longer[9].

YOU'LL ENJOY FISH AT LEAST TWICE A WEEK

As well as being protein-rich, fish and seafood are full of nutrients that help to keep our metabolism humming.

YOU'LL GET AT LEAST THREE DAILY SERVINGS OF NUTRITIOUS CARBOHYDRATES (WHICH INCLUDE WHOLEGRAINS)

YOU'LL EAT THREE SERVINGS OF DAIRY FOODS DAILY

Dairy foods not only brim with bone-building calcium and protein but studies suggest that a regular dairy and calcium intake can give weight loss a boost – possibly by cutting fat absorption and controlling appetite. One US study[10] found that consuming three servings a day of calcium-rich dairy foods as part of a calorie-controlled diet boosted weight loss by 70%, compared to those on a standard calorie-controlled diet. If you don't eat dairy foods, choose calcium-fortified soya milk and soya yogurts instead.

YOU'LL GET PLENTY OF FIBRE

Weight loss has been found to be an amazing *three times* greater for people eating high-fibre, low-fat diets compared with low-fat alone[11]. Fibre seems to help by boosting the feeling of satisfaction we get after eating. Fibre-rich foods tend to take longer to chew, digest and absorb – which in turn gives our body's appetite messengers more time to work and let us know when we're full. We get fibre from high-fibre cereals, wholegrains, pulses, vegetables, fruit, nuts and seeds.

YOU'LL EMBRACE HEALTHY FATS

Don't be afraid of fat! We all need some in our daily diet and this plan includes vital mood-boosting omega-3s (a happy slimmer is a more successful slimmer, as there's no need for comfort eating when you're smiling!) and healthy unsaturated fats, while limiting cholesterol-raising saturated and trans fats.

▶ WHAT ABOUT CAFFEINE?

I used to drink about two litres (3½ pints) of coffee a day and felt permanently nauseous as a result. Then I swapped to decaffeinated black tea and green tea and experienced an incredible boost to my wellbeing. Lyndel says that some people are very sensitive to caffeine (it can make them feel jittery or get headaches), and feel best when they avoid or limit it. She also says that other people are fine having it, and even find it beneficial when enjoyed in moderation (up to two to three cups daily of brewed coffee or five to six cups of tea).

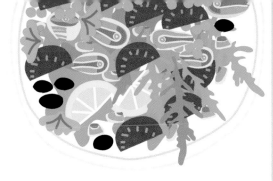

THE *ADORE YOURSELF SLIM* EATING PLAN

The *Adore Yourself Slim* Eating Plan provides about 1,400–1,500 calories daily, but there's no need to get bogged down by counting calories as Lyndel's done that for you. However, it can help to know that to lose a healthy 1lb (0.5kg) over a week you need to eat about 500 fewer calories each day than your body currently needs.

■ There's no set length of time for you to follow the weight-loss phase of the eating plan. The important thing is to be realistic about how quickly and how much weight you want to lose. Realistic goals

> ❝ **Unrealistic goals are a slap to your self-esteem. Realistic goals are achievable, and success boosts your confidence to continue** ❞

are achievable, and success boosts your confidence to continue. Unrealistic goals are a sure-fire route to failure and a slap to your self-esteem. Remember, too, that a great target to aim for is to lose 5–10% of your bodyweight (see page 49) – you can always lose more later on if you want to.

■ 'We know from research[4,12] that when people decide to make changes to their eating and/or exercise habits, they lose the most weight over three to six months,' says Lyndel. 'After that, things tend to level off a bit – or you may even regain some weight, largely because it's so easy to lose your focus. If this happens, then plenty of help is at hand (see Chapter 6: Get Yourself Over A Plateau, pages 116–121). You may find that

three months is a good length of time to be actively losing weight. Then have a rest, and keep up the basics of your new approach for a few months while deciding if you want to go on to lose a bit more.' Once you've reached a weight you're happy with, you can go on to our Stay Slim Plan (see page 140), which, although you're allowed a few extra servings of food each day, will help you to maintain your new weight.

■ The *Adore Yourself Slim* Eating Plan uses a simple food-swap system. This means you can choose foods you enjoy and that best suit your lifestyle. It's flexible, but still fairly structured. However, to keep this eating plan balanced, it's important to eat the recommended number of servings from each food group every day. If you eat a bit more one day – you will, life happens – then no worries, just aim to cut back a bit the next day so that you're in balance over a few days.

■ It's definitely worth weighing or measuring out some of the foods once or twice, as serving sizes may be bigger or smaller than you're used to. Research[13] suggests that we can eat up to 25% less at a meal before our body notices the difference. Try eating from smaller plates and bowls.

■ At each meal, aim to combine a feel-full-for-longer-for-fewer-calories combination of lean protein-rich foods (this includes dairy foods) and plenty of veg or salad (at least half your plate) and/or fruit.

THE *ADORE YOURSELF SLIM* EATING PLAN AT A GLANCE

It's as easy as 1, 2, 3!

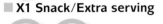

■ **X1 Snack/Extra serving**

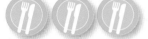

■ **X2 Fruit servings**

■ **X3 Protein servings**
■ **X3 Nutritious Carbohydrates servings**
■ **X3 Dairy servings**
■ **X3 Fat servings**

■ **Unlimited vegetables and salad**
■ **Condiments**
■ **Drinks**

GENERAL GUIDELINES
■ Ideally, limit red meat to three or four times a week. Eat fish at least twice a week, and include oily fish.
■ There's no need to limit eggs, unless you've been advised to by your doctor.
■ Aim to include pulses, nuts or seeds on most days of the week.
■ Men and very active women should add one Nutritious Carbohydrates serving, plus one extra Fat and one extra Dairy or Snack/Extra serving (ideally not as alcohol!) each day.

WHAT LISA ATE FOOD	NUMBER OF SERVINGS
Breakfast 6 heaped tbsp muesli with 150ml (5fl oz) skimmed milk and two handfuls of frozen berries	1 Fruit, 2 Nutritious Carbohydrates, ½ Dairy
Snack Handful of nuts plus 2 kiwi fruit	1 Snack/Extra, 1 Fruit
Lunch 2 slices of ham on a slice of wholegrain rye bread plus a big green salad dressed with 1 tsp olive oil and balsamic vinegar	1 Protein, 1 Nutritious Carbohydrates, 1 Fat, Vegetables
Snack ½ pot low-fat pineapple cottage cheese	1 Dairy
Dinner Stir-fry made with 150g (5½oz) chicken breast, lots of veg and spices and 2 tsp oil, plus a low-fat fruit bioyogurt	2 Protein, 1 Dairy, 2 Fat, Vegetables
Throughout the day 150ml (5fl oz) skimmed milk in tea, plus lots of green and herbal tea, plus 1 litre (1¾ pints) water	½ Dairy, 8 Drinks

YOUR QUESTIONS ANSWERED

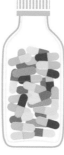

Is the eating plan suitable for my whole family?

This eating plan has been put together for adults (those over 18), but the variety of foods and meals you make up from them, including the recipes, are a suitable basis for the whole family. It's best for partners, children and other family members who don't need to lose weight to add more Nutritious Carbohydrates (such as bread, pasta, rice or potatoes) to their meals – an ideal balance on their plate would be one-third Protein, one-third veg or salad and one-third Nutritious Carbohydrates. Meal sizes will be proportionally smaller for children, according to how much you might normally serve them (remember, too, that children under five have different nutritional needs to older children).

What if I'm vegetarian or vegan?

You can still follow the *Adore Yourself Slim* Eating Plan. Vegetarian foods from the Protein list include eggs, pulses (split peas, beans, lentils, chickpeas), tofu, Quorn, nuts and seeds. Dairy products are also suitable. If you're vegan, then pulses, tofu/other soya products, nuts and seeds will be your key Protein foods, and calcium-fortified soya milk, cheese and yogurt will replace foods from the Dairy group.

Will I need to take a vitamin and mineral supplement?

'You can use a variety of foods from all the key food groups to create your eating plan so that it can be nutritious and balanced,' says Lyndel. 'However, people often like to take a one-a-day multivitamin and mineral supplement (with amounts close to the RDA) as an insurance policy, especially when they're slimming, as they're eating less overall. This is particularly wise if you're vegetarian or vegan to ensure that your nutrient needs are met (for example, vitamin B12 is only naturally found in meat, dairy foods and eggs).

> **❝ Take a one-a-day multivitamin and mineral supplement as an insurance policy when slimming as you're eating less overall ❞**

▶ LISA'S TOP TIP

When I followed eating plans in the past, I found the thing that really put me off was having to eat 21 different meals a week – it was just too daunting to get my head around. So when I developed my own eating plan, I ate more or less the same kind of meal every day to start with, for example porridge for breakfast; a different salad with protein for lunch; and protein with veggies for dinner; plus yogurt, cottage cheese or nuts as snacks. When Lyndel revised my plan, I was relieved when she said that it's fine to eat more or less the same kind of meals every day initially to keep things simple, and then, when you feel more confident about the plan and know it off by heart, to start consulting the food lists and swapping in interesting alternatives.

THE *ADORE YOURSELF SLIM* FOOD LISTS

SNACKS/EXTRAS
1 serving is…

- 1 palmful of nuts or seeds
- 1 oatcake spread thinly with nut butter/ hummus plus cherry tomatoes
- ½ medium avocado
- 1 large banana
- 150g (5½oz) pot low-fat rice pudding
- 1 boiled egg plus 1 apple or 2 brown rice cakes
- 2 oatcakes or 3 brown rice cakes thinly spread with light soft cheese
- 1 light cheese triangle plus sliced carrot, celery and red pepper
- 125g (4½oz) (½ x average pot) low-fat cottage cheese (plain or flavoured) with carrot sticks
- 28g (1oz) popcorn, popped with ½ tsp oil
- 28g (1oz) or 3 squares dark chocolate (or other favourite snack containing about 130 cals)
- 125ml (4fl oz) wine* (1.5 units of alcohol) or 285ml (½ pint)/1 small bottle of beer or cider (1-1.5 units of alcohol) or 25-35ml (1-1¼fl oz) measure of spirits (1-1.5 units of alcohol) plus low-calorie mixer
- 1 extra Nutritious Carbohydrates serving

FRUIT
1 serving is…

- 1 medium piece of fruit (apple, pear, orange, peach, nectarine, banana)
- 2 small fruit (satsumas, plums, kiwi fruit, figs – fresh or dried)
- ½ grapefruit or 14 cherries or 6 lychees
- 3 heaped tbsp canned fruit in natural juice
- 2 large 5cm (2in) thick slices of mango
- 1 large 5cm (2in) thick slice of melon, pineapple or papaya
- 2 handfuls of berries (fresh or frozen)
- 3 apricots (fresh or dried) or prunes
- 1 heaped tbsp raisins, currants or sultanas

PROTEIN
1 serving is…

- 75g (2¾oz) raw weight (roughly the size of your palm) lean beef, pork, lamb, chicken, turkey or oily fish (see page 71 for a list)
- 2 medium slices (about 75g/2¾oz) of lean cooked meat (roast beef, pork, turkey, chicken, pork, ham)
- 100g (3½oz) (raw weight; chequebook-sized) non-oily white fish (see page 71 for a list)
- 100g (3½oz) seafood (see page 71 for a list)
- 85g (3oz) can or ½ x 185-200g (6½-7oz) can tuna in brine, spring water or non-oily sauce
- 3 canned sardines or ½ x 125g (4½oz) can mackerel or ¼ x 425g (15oz) can pilchards in brine, spring water or non-oily sauce
- 105g (3¾oz) or ½ x 213g (7½oz) can salmon
- 2 small or medium eggs
- 2 tbsp hummus
- 4 heaped tbsp cooked/ canned kidney, butter, soya or other beans, baked beans, split peas, lentils or chickpeas (but you can have unlimited amounts of mange tout and canned, fresh or frozen green beans – see Unlimited Vegetables And Salad, opposite)
- Bowl (about 300ml/ ½ pint) of lentil/bean and vegetable soup
- 100g (3½oz) original or smoked tofu or Quorn (pieces or mince) or 50g (1¾oz) marinated tofu
- 28g (1oz) seeds or nuts (about 2 rounded tbsp) or 2 level tbsp peanut butter

NUTRITIOUS CARBOHYDRATES

1 serving is…

- 40g (1½oz) or about 5 tbsp wholegrain or bran-based cereal or porridge oats
- 2 Shredded Wheat or Weetabix
- 40g (1½oz) or 3 heaped tbsp muesli
- 1 medium slice of wholegrain, wholemeal, pumpernickel, rye, spelt or Granary bread
- 1 mini pita or tortilla or ½ medium pita or tortilla (preferably wholemeal)
- 2 oatcakes or 3 rye crackers
- ½ cup cooked (28g/1oz uncooked) brown or basmati rice, soba or egg noodles, wholewheat pasta or quinoa
- ½ jacket potato or 2 egg-sized potatoes
- 100g (3½oz) or 1 medium sweet potato
- 3 heaped tbsp cooked/canned kidney, butter, soya or other beans, baked beans, split peas, lentils or chickpeas (but you can have unlimited amounts of mange tout and canned, fresh or frozen green beans – see Unlimited Vegetables And Salad, below right)
- 4 heaped tbsp garden peas, mushy peas or processed peas
- 5 heaped tbsp petit pois
- 1 corn cob or 3 heaped tbsp canned or frozen sweetcorn kernels

DAIRY

This list also includes Dairy alternatives.

1 serving is…

- 300ml (½ pint) skimmed milk
- 200ml (7fl oz) semi-skimmed milk or calcium-fortified soya milk
- Small pot (about 125g/4½oz) low-fat fruit bioyogurt or soya yogurt
- 150g (5½oz) pot or 4 tbsp natural yogurt
- 28g (1oz) firm cheese: preferably opt for medium-fat cheeses that contain up to 29g fat per 100g (3½oz), such as Edam, Gouda, Jarlsburg, Brie, Camembert, Parmesan, goat's cheese, feta, halloumi and reduced-fat Cheddar. High-fat cheeses (more than 29g fat per 100g/ 3½oz) include Danish Blue, Saint Agur, full-fat Cheddar and Comté – have these less often
- 50g (1¾oz) light soft cheese
- 125g (4½oz) (½ x average pot) low-fat cottage cheese (plain or flavoured)

FATS

1 serving is…

- 1 tsp oil (extra-virgin olive, rapeseed, walnut, peanut/groundnut or toasted sesame)
- 1 tsp butter or olive oil- or rapeseed oil-based spread
- 4 tbsp gravy made with granules and hot water only
- 1 tsp mayonnaise
- 2 tsp salad dressing or salad cream
- 1 tsp peanut butter, tahini, seeds or nuts

UNLIMITED VEGETABLES AND SALAD

- Eat *at least* four servings a day and include plenty with your lunch and dinner.
- Choose freely, but remember that certain vegetables, such as avocados, sweet potatoes, potatoes, sweetcorn, corn, canned beans (excluding green beans), peas, petit pois, split peas, chickpeas and lentils, do need to be measured out, as they're more calorific than most other vegetables.

CONDIMENTS

■ See The Savvy Shopper's Food Shopping List, opposite, for a list of spices, herbs and condiments.

■ With olives, limit yourself to four to six per meal (but the good news is, you don't have to count them as part of any of your servings).

■ As brown, tomato and sweet chilli sauce all contain quite a bit of sugar, limit them to 2 teaspoons per day.

■ As this eating plan is based on fresh rather than processed foods, it'll keep your salt intake in check. However, olives, most sauces and pickled foods are salty, so use them sparingly and aim not to add extra salt when cooking.

DRINKS

■ Have at least eight glasses or cups of fluid over the day (that's at least 1.6 litres/2¾ pints), or more if you're very active or it's hot. If your urine is light straw coloured, then you're drinking enough. If it's dark, then drink more. Choose from water (tap, mineral or sparkling, soda); tea (black, green, redbush, herbal, fruit or ginger infusions); coffee.

■ If you have milk in drinks, or a milky coffee, use milk from your Dairy allocation.

■ Avoid sugary drinks. Limit sugar-free 'diet' drinks to rare treats rather than daily drinks – they're usually full of unhelpful additives and sweeteners, and some contain caffeine.

■*Remember wise drinking. To keep any risks to your health low, NHS advice is that women should not exceed 2–3 units of alcohol per day (for men it's 3–4 units) on a regular basis. 25ml spirits, 285ml (½ pint) standard beer/lager/cider or 90ml wine contains 1 unit (125ml wine contains about 1.5 units, and 175ml about 2 units). Those planning to conceive or who are pregnant are advised to avoid drinking alcohol.

> **❝The wise man should consider that health is the greatest of human blessings. Let food be your medicine ❞**
> *Hippocrates*

THE SAVVY SHOPPER'S FOOD SHOPPING LIST

Now it's time to perform what I call a Kitchen Cleanse – clear out all the foods that were part of your old, non-nurturing lifestyle and restock your kitchen cupboards, freezer and fridge with these healthy ingredients. Take this book with you the first time you go on an *Adore Yourself Slim* food-shopping outing and tick off the storecupboard ingredients as you buy them. I suggest you get everything you think you'll ever need all at once if you can. If you're unable to find all the condiments or spices listed here in a single shop or supermarket, make it your mission to track them down and give yourself a deadline for doing so. As this list includes every single item mentioned in both the *Adore Yourself Slim* Eating Plan and the Stay Slim Plan (including the recipes on pages 85–93), this will mean you'll never not be able to cook healthy food again because you're missing a vital ingredient. On future trips, take photocopies of this list so that you'll know what additional fresh items you need to buy – and what you've already got in your cupboard, fridge or freezer at home. Get set for a culinary adventure...

CONDIMENTS, SEASONINGS, SAUCES, SPREADS AND OILS

Black peppercorns
Cayenne pepper
Salt
Caraway seeds
Bouquet garni sachets
Ground turmeric/cinnamon/ginger
Cumin seeds
Dried thyme/chives/bay leaves/cloves
Curry powder/paste
Gravy granules
Stock cubes
Chilli flakes/fresh chillies
Garlic (fresh, paste, granules)
Fresh root ginger
Fresh parsley/basil/coriander
Mustard (wholegrain, English, Dijon)/mustard powder
Wasabi/horseradish sauce
Lime pickle
Thai fish sauce/soy sauce
Sauce (brown, Worcestershire, tomato, sweet chilli, chilli, hot pepper)
Teriyaki marinade
Vinegar (balsamic, red wine, malt)

Mayonnaise/salad dressing/salad cream

Oil (extra-virgin olive, rapeseed, walnut, peanut/groundnut, toasted sesame)

Peanut butter/nut butter/tahini

Bovril/Marmite

CANNED/BOTTLED GOODS

Salsa

Sun-dried tomatoes

Capers

Anchovies

Olives, including Kalamata

Chopped canned tomatoes

Tomato purée

Peppadews/pickled onions/gherkins/pickled cucumbers/pickled vegetables

Canned beans (kidney, butter, green, soya, baked beans, adzuki, cannellini, haricot)

Chickpeas/peas/mushy peas/processed peas/sweetcorn

Sardines/mackerel/pilchards in brine, spring water or non-oily sauce

Salmon

Tuna in brine, spring water or non-oily sauce

Canned fruit in natural juice

MISCELLANEOUS

Plain flour/cornflour

Honey

Low-sugar fruit jam/marmalade

Stem ginger in syrup

Currants/raisins/sultanas

Dried figs/other dried fruit

Seeds (sesame, pumpkin, linseed, sunflower)

Omega-3 seed sprinkles/mixed unsalted nuts/pine nuts/peanuts

Porridge oats/muesli/wholegrain and bran-based breakfast cereals

Bread (rye, wholegrain, wholemeal, Granary, pumpernickel, spelt);
wholemeal pita bread/tortillas

Popcorn

Oatcakes/rye crackers/brown rice cakes

Soba or egg noodles/wholewheat pasta

Dried beans/lentils/split peas

Quinoa

Brown or basmati rice

Good-quality dark chocolate (70% cocoa solids)

Tea (black/green/redbush/herbal/fruit/ginger infusions)/coffee

Sparkling water/mineral water/soda water (tap water is fine too!)/
low-calorie mixers

FRESH FOODS

Lemons/limes

Fresh fruit

Fresh vegetables

Potatoes/sweet potatoes

Salad leaves/salad ingredients/avocados

FROZEN AND REFRIGERATED FOODS

Semi-skimmed and skimmed milk/soya milk

Seafood (prawns, shrimps, calamari, crab, mussels, oysters, squid)

Non-oily white fish (haddock, pollock, cod, plaice, coley)

Oily fish (smoked and fresh salmon, sardines, smoked and fresh mackerel, trout,
pilchards, Arctic char, fresh tuna, herring, kippers, eel, whitebait)

Cooked meats (beef, pork, ham, turkey, chicken)/Parma ham/prosciutto

Fresh lean beef/pork/lamb/chicken/turkey

Frozen vegetables (peas, spinach, petit pois, green beans, soya beans, edamame,
cauliflower, broccoli, sweetcorn, etc)

Frozen berries

Eggs (standard or omega-3 enriched)

Tofu/Quorn

Natural low-fat bioyogurt/fruit bioyogurt/soya yogurt

Low-fat cottage cheese (plain or flavoured)/light soft cheese/
light cheese triangles

Medium-fat firm cheese (any with up to 29g fat per 100g/3½oz)

High-fat firm cheese (any with over 29g fat per 100g/3½oz)

Butter/olive oil- or rapeseed oil-based spread

Standard or reduced-fat hummus

Low-fat rice pudding

ITEMS FROM THE *ADORE YOURSELF SLIM* STAY SLIM PLAN

Ice cream/low-fat custard

Fruit juice/smoothies

Pesto

Your own Sanity Savers (see page 72)

7 SANITY SAVERS

These are the snacks that'll keep you on track when hunger – whether real, imagined or emotion driven – kicks in. I swear by the ones below, but you're bound to have your own, so write them down in the space provided and add to your list as you discover more.

1 Soup Low-cal homemade vegetable soup is a great hole filler (especially during that hungry hour before your evening meal) or as a starter[14]. French research[15] reveals that regular veg-based soup eaters tend to be not only slimmer but have better intakes of key vitamins, too.

2 A handful of frozen berries
These are a great standby for when you feel like something sweet. Enjoy them as mini ice lollies straight from the freezer, or allow them to thaw and top with a spoonful of fruit yogurt (served in a martini glass, this also makes an impressive-looking dessert).

3 A couple of handfuls of raw veggies
Craving crisps? Crunching on sliced carrots, mange tout, peppers and cherry tomatoes will stop you caving in. Keep some chopped up in a sealed container in the fridge and serve with salsa or a yogurt-based dip.

4 Cooked apple with cinnamon
When I'm prowling the house looking for the chocolate I know isn't there, this is my favourite Sanity Saver. Simply cook a chopped-up apple with 2 tbsp water and a sprinkling of ground cinnamon (which is said to help stabilise your blood-sugar levels) for a sweet treat that'll stop you heading for the corner shop.

5 Olives, soya beans and tofu A handful of four to six juicy Kalamata olives while cooking is enough to keep my appetite in check until dinner's ready. A small handful of cooked soya beans or cubes of smoked tofu with sesame seeds also does the trick.

6 Exotic fruit A small tub of chopped-up fruit in the fridge – think mango, pineapple, oranges, kiwi – makes a scrumptious choice in a need-to-nibble emergency. Keep the tub sealed to lock in precious antioxidants.

7 A small portion of your favourite food Successful slimmers don't view any foods as truly forbidden. Instead, they show *flexible restraint* by occasionally enjoying a small amount of their favourite foods as part of a healthy diet. Sometimes your daily Snack/Extra option (see page 66) will be enough, but at other times enjoying some of your favourite food (no matter how fattening it is) is a Sanity Saver because it helps you feel satisfied and avoid all-or-nothing/'What-the-heck' thinking. I encourage my hypnotherapy patients to schedule in a treat meal or indulgent snack regularly so they don't feel that they're depriving themselves, just delaying the pleasure a little. Food you've really been looking forward to always tastes that little bit nicer. List your own Sanity Savers below.

THE TOP SLIMMING FOODS

There is no magic wand when it comes to weight loss, but the benefits of some foods and drinks could just add up to give your body the little boost it needs to help you get more rewarding results.

1 GREEN TEA

The philosopher Bernard-Paul Heroux once famously said: 'There is no trouble so great or grave that cannot be much diminished by a nice cup of tea.' Interestingly, it's also true that waistline 'trouble' could be 'much diminished' by regularly drinking green tea. A review of studies[16] found that the combination of caffeine and catechins (antioxidants) in green tea can increase energy expenditure (calories burned), while another review[17] linked green tea to modest weight loss.

2 CHILLI

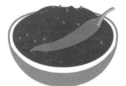

Chilli adds tantalizing flavour to food, and has been shown[18] to boost metabolic rate briefly and help manage hunger. Enjoy chilli in cooking – think healthy curries, chilli con carne, fragrant Thai soups and salads.

3 BEANS

Beans help you to feel fuller for longer thanks to their fibre content. This seems due to their effect on a hormone called cholecystokinin (CCK), which works as a natural appetite suppressant by slowing down how quickly your stomach empties. Researchers at the University of California[19] found that levels of CCK were twice as high after a meal containing beans than after a low-fibre meal without them.

4 EGGS

Eggs are the ultimate fast food. When I'm seeing a patient in the evening and literally have only five minutes to cook, I grab whatever I can (mushrooms, onion, peppers, baby tomatoes, canned tuna, prawns, capers) and throw it in a frying pan along with two beaten eggs. Served with a handful of baby spinach dressed with balsamic vinegar, it's a filling meal in minutes. Eggs have slimming superpowers, too: a US study[20] found that overweight women who had two eggs for breakfast on five or more days a week for two months as part of a low-fat diet lost an

❝ A study has shown that having a big salad with a low-fat dressing before a meal could help you eat about 100 calories less overall during that meal ❞

incredible 65% more weight than participants who ate a bagel breakfast with the same number of calories.

5 SALAD

Yeah, we all know salad is good for us. But have a big salad before a meal (with a low-fat dressing) and it could help you eat about 100 calories less overall during that meal. That's what happened to women taking part in a study at Penn State University[21], even though they were offered as much pasta as they wanted after the salad. I simply adore a colourful salad for lunch. To the basics (baby spinach, baby tomatoes, cucumber, red pepper) I add different tasty ingredients (canned tuna, sprouted beans, Peppadews, olives, feta cheese, onion, Parma ham, gherkins) and am always surprised at how wonderfully full I feel, even without having any bread with it.

THE TEN SLIMMING COMMANDMENTS

1 THOU SHALT NOT ORDER SUSHI IF THOU DOESN'T LIKE FISH

A cardinal rule of this programme is to only eat food you adore. I used to make the mistake of eating floppy yellowing broccoli along with a piece of freezer-burned chicken and then wonder why I found it so hard to slim. On this programme, you may not be able to eat *whatever* you like all the time (we're practising flexible restraint, remember), but it's a non-negotiable rule to eat *only* what you like!

2 THOU SHALT BARGE TO THE FRONT OF YOUR OWN QUEUE

When you're slimming, you need to put yourself first. Nothing is more important than eating well and exercising, because if you don't have good health and feel good about yourself, you can't make the most of everything life has to offer – or be there for the people who need you. Ask yourself daily, 'What do I need to do today to stay on track?' and make that your first priority.

3 THOU SHALT EAT SLOWLY AND STOP WHEN YOU'RE COMFORTABLY FULL (NOT STUFFED)

People who eat quickly are twice as likely to be overweight as those who don't, according to a recent Japanese study[22]. Eating slowly is a great way to give yourself time to register that you're full as it allows appetite-regulating messages from your stomach to your brain to build up to optimal levels.

4 THOU SHALT ASK YOURSELF, 'WHAT DO I *REALLY* NEED RIGHT NOW?'

Ask yourself this all-important question every time you want to eat outside your designated meal and snack times, and you'll often be surprised by the answer. It took me 20 years to realise that when I get ravenously hungry just before bedtime, it's because I actually need to sleep, not rev up my tired body with a sugar boost so that I can stay awake longer. If you're truly hungry, make a choice based on what you really feel like eating, preferably from your eating plan or a Sanity Saver (see page 72). But the rest of the time, stop, think and give your body what it's actually asking for – a break, a glass of water or a hug.

5 THOU SHALT NEVER EAT ANYTHING BIGGER THAN YOUR HEAD

I was always terrified of being hungry, so I used to eat huge meals. Even when I ate

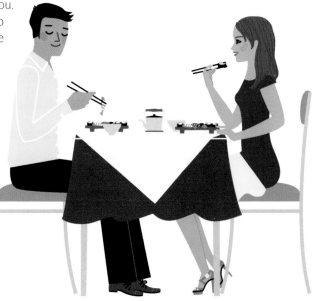

healthily, my family-sized, serves-six salad bowl would elicit amazed comments from my colleagues. Then one day it dawned on me that my failure to lose weight wasn't just about *what* I ate but also about *how much* I ate. So I swapped my crater-sized bowl for a non-super-sized one, but promised myself second helpings should this mini-meal not be enough. And to my astonishment, I found that I felt pleasantly full on a lot less food.

6 THOU SHALT REPEAT AFTER ME: 'EVERY LITTLE BIT HELPS'

You didn't become overweight in a day, and you're not going to slim down in one either. It took thousands of tiny lifestyle decisions to get you where you are today, and by the same token, many tiny lifestyle decisions are going to help you slim. Think about every bite of food you take, think about every move you make and ask yourself, 'Is there any way I can turn this into an opportunity to adore myself slim?' Little by little those calories you shave off here and there and those extra bits of energy expenditure are going to add up to a lovely surprise on the scales.

7 THOU SHALT REMEMBER WHAT'S IN IT FOR YOU

Make the reasons that you're slimming mouthwateringly, spine-tinglingly appealing (see page 45). It's hard to get excited about losing weight to avoid heart disease (though you'll no doubt be very grateful for this value-added benefit later in life), but easy to get your heart aflutter at the thought of fitting into that adorable dress you've been eyeing up, or having more energy and confidence. Psychologists have found that focusing on things other than just appearance means we're more likely to succeed at slimming in the long term.

8 THOU SHALT FORGIVE AND FORGET

Just because you caved in and ate a whole packet of biscuits for breakfast doesn't mean that's a reason to feel a failure and pig out for the rest of the day (or week). Punishing yourself for a lapse by bingeing on unhealthy food until your conscience kicks in is a sure-fire way to sabotage your weight loss. Instead, dust off those crumbs, say 'I forgive myself' and get back on the wagon right away. See a setback as an opportunity to plan how you might act differently in the future (use the *Adore Yourself Slim* Travel Journal on page 148 to help you do this).

9 THOU SHALT REMEMBER THAT IF YOU FAIL TO PLAN, YOU PLAN TO FAIL

I used to live on ready-meals as I thought I was too busy to shop for fresh produce. Now I religiously go shopping for my week's worth of salad and vegetables on a Monday because I know that if I don't start the week right, I'm doomed to wander off track. And I diarise all my exercise sessions and fit in other commitments around them, not the other way round.

10 THOU SHALT LEARN TO RELAX

Numerous studies[23] have shown that stress can make you fat, and as hypnosis is a form of deep relaxation, this is one of the reasons why it's such an effective slimming tool (so don't forget to listen to your hypnosis CD twice a day). Remember, rest and sleep are just as vital as activity in helping to shift the pounds. Research[24] shows that regular sleep deprivation puts hormones that regulate appetite and metabolism (such as leptin, cortisol and insulin) out of whack, which can lead to food cravings and weight gain.

HOW TO HANDLE HUNGER AND CRAVINGS

If you ever find yourself craving food even though you've recently eaten, then you know you're not eating just because you're hungry. Rather, an emotion or situation has triggered the habitual response of using food to feel better or treat yourself. Because this 'non-hungry' eating is usually a learned behaviour, you can unlearn it and reprogramme the way you react to the things that trigger it. Once you've finished reading this chapter, the hypnosis track you'll listen to will also help you do this. Now read more about the different types of hunger and cravings, and ideas for dealing with them…

TYPE OF HUNGER	HOW TO DEAL WITH IT
Real hunger occurs as a result of the interaction between a number of hormones and a fall in blood sugar that signal the need to refuel by eating. We gradually become aware of an emptiness in our stomach and may experience a rumbling tummy, an uneasiness and light-headedness. This feeling quickly passes when we eat.	Eating at regular intervals will help regulate hunger (see page 61). But of course, we all know that hunger isn't the only trigger for eating. The hunger scale below will help you to recognise if you're *physically hungry* or eating for *other* reasons. When you get the urge to eat in between meals or when you've finished your planned meal, stop and assess how truly hungry you feel using the scale.

❝Avoid feeling stuffed or very hungry as this can trigger overeating❞

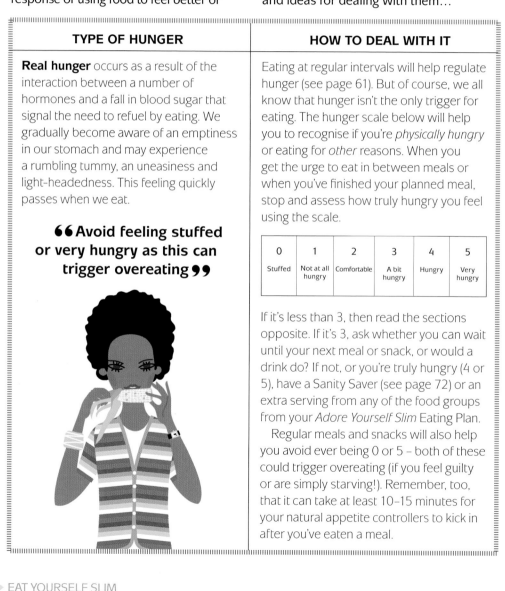

0	1	2	3	4	5
Stuffed	Not at all hungry	Comfortable	A bit hungry	Hungry	Very hungry

If it's less than 3, then read the sections opposite. If it's 3, ask whether you can wait until your next meal or snack, or would a drink do? If not, or you're truly hungry (4 or 5), have a Sanity Saver (see page 72) or an extra serving from any of the food groups from your *Adore Yourself Slim* Eating Plan.

Regular meals and snacks will also help you avoid ever being 0 or 5 – both of these could trigger overeating (if you feel guilty or are simply starving!). Remember, too, that it can take at least 10–15 minutes for your natural appetite controllers to kick in after you've eaten a meal.

TYPE OF HUNGER	HOW TO DEAL WITH IT
Emotional hunger is the type that often causes 'non-hungry' eating. It can develop quickly in response to an emotion or feeling and is usually experienced as an intense craving for food, or an 'empty' feeling. Eating brings initial relief, but you may feel guilty or 'bad' soon afterwards.	Before you eat, think HALT, asking yourself, 'Am I Hungry, Angry, Lonely or Tired? What do I *really* need right now?' If you are truly Hungry, eat (see Real Hunger, opposite). If you're Angry, think of strategies to resolve the situation; if you're Lonely, call someone; if you're Tired, can you rest? Seek professional help if you think your emotions are too difficult to deal with on your own.
Bored hunger occurs, for example, when you've been sitting at your desk all morning or in front of the TV all evening and get a sudden urge to splurge on something sugary, salty or fat-laden, such as biscuits, crisps or chocolate.	This is a sign that your brain is craving variety, not a wedge of cake! Distract yourself by having a cup of tea or glass of water, doing a Sneaky Workout (see page 99), changing your work task, painting or filing your nails or going for a walk. If you're often at a loose end at home, consider signing up for evening or dance classes or doing some voluntary work.
Stressed hunger is the kind you tend to experience when you're burning the candle at both ends. You're permanently exhausted and feel you need to continuously refuel yourself to keep going. Stress hunger is a double whammy because when you're stressed you feel too busy to exercise, so you eat more and exercise less.	Vigorous exercise to burn off the adrenalin coursing through your body is the quickest way to de-stress during or after a stressful day. Another fantastic calming technique is to breathe in to the count of four through your nose, pause and then breathe out again through your nose to the count of eight. Focus on releasing any unnecessary nervous tension in your body while breathing out. Hypnosis works a treat, too.
Cravings are an intense desire to eat a particular (usually sugary or high-fat) food. While it may feel as if they just randomly pop into your head, they're usually the result of some form of trigger – a thought or emotion, or the smell or sight of food that you spot in the supermarket, a magazine or on TV.	Like waves, cravings build up and then ebb away after about 10–15 minutes. An effective way to deal with them is to 'surf' them. Talk yourself through it: 'I don't *really* need to eat. This craving is a learned habit that will soon pass.' The more you successfully 'surf', the weaker the link between a trigger and craving becomes.

SANITY-SAVING STRATEGIES

You can't stop going out or interacting with others while you're losing weight (or when keeping it off), but social situations and other people can often divert you from your mission to adore yourself slim. Occasionally you will no doubt want to say 'Yes' to treats (see Sanity Savers on page 72), but for those other times, when saying 'No' is the best way forward, here are some tried-and-tested strategies that are useful in helping to avoid or limit fattening foods without causing offence or sounding like a diet bore.

WHAT TO SAY WHEN…

Your mother-in-law/a friend offers you a piece of pie that she's spent all morning baking. You don't really fancy it, but are worried you'll upset her if you refuse it.
It can be hard when you feel you're upsetting others or refusing love or friendship, but remember that you're entitled to be the one who decides what and how much you eat, and to put your needs first. It can take practice to feel comfortable saying 'No, thank you' or 'Just a very small piece, please', so take time to try it out first at home, by yourself. Another tactic you could try is to say, 'Thanks so much for going to so much trouble, but I'm really too full to have any. Perhaps I'll have some later.' Then 'forget' to ask for some.

Cream cake is being passed around your workplace to celebrate someone's birthday and you really want some.
This depends on the type of person you are. If you can't stop once you've said 'Yes', simply say: 'I had a late lunch/I'm really full right now/I may have some later.' However, if you feel you can have some and still remain in control, say 'I'm really not that hungry (even if you are!), so I'll have a very small piece.' (You only need to mention you're slimming if you feel like doing so.) Then have the smallest slice you can cut off and savour every last crumb. Food eaten in this way tastes exquisite. It's also helpful to suggest that more healthy alternatives, such as strawberries or crudités with dips, are served alongside celebration cakes in future – others will probably thank you for requesting an alternative.

You've been invited to dinner at a friend's and you're afraid the food will scupper your healthy-eating plans.
Be honest and tell your friend in advance that you've adopted a healthier lifestyle and so would be grateful if she/he'd serve plenty of veggies or salad (that way, even if the main course is really calorific you'll be able to fill most of your plate with low-cal veggies; you'll also avoid sounding like a fussy eater). Remember, if it makes you feel awkward, you don't need to mention you're slimming.

Your colleagues are forever offering to fetch you sweet treats from the canteen, vending machine or corner shop.
Your close colleagues are the people you spend most time with, so it's hard to hide the fact that you're slimming or eating more healthily from them. If you do decide to tell, ask them to support your efforts. However, if you decide not to inform your colleagues, and don't feel strong enough to say 'No, thanks', be prepared to do some serious fibbing: 'I'm not in the mood for anything sweet today,' and 'I've just eaten' are both believable excuses.

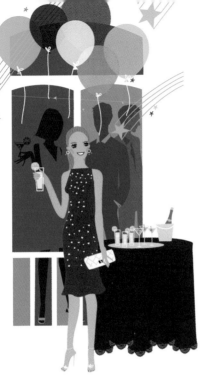

THE LOOK-AHEAD LIST

Life doesn't go on hold when you're slimming, so you need to be prepared when things get stressful or you experience changes to your routine. Some of these ideas will help...

WHAT TO DO WHEN...
You forget your packed lunch and have only a corner shop or service station to buy from.
- ■ Any sandwich or salad with 350 calories.
- ■ 50g (1¾oz) packet of nuts; a piece of fruit.

You get home late, feeling shattered and starving hungry.
- ■ Keep a stock of healthy ready-meals (based on meat, chicken, fish, prawns or pulses) in the freezer. Choose ones with up to 400 calories and serve with steamed veg (ready-prepared fresh or frozen) or salad.

You have an early appointment and don't get up in time to eat breakfast.
- ■ A cereal bar (about 130 calories) with a mini cheese and piece of fruit.
- ■ Before leaving home, spread a wholegrain roll or sandwich with peanut butter or fill it with a slice of cold meat and some salad.

You're on your way to the gym and feeling hungry.
- ■ A banana or mini fruit bun.
- ■ A cereal bar or pot of rice pudding.

You're invited to a meal in a restaurant.
Offer to play an active role in researching the restaurants you're considering going to by looking up their menu online or calling them to ensure that they cater for your new way of eating. If you don't have any say in where you go, become what I call a Slimming Detective and seek out crafty ways to make a meal as healthy as possible (order a soup or salad starter; skip bread; avoid creamy sauces and fried foods; ask for any dressings or sauces on the side; share a dessert, etc).

You're invited to a family celebration.
- ■ Have a bowl of soup, a salad or a snack from your Dairy serving list before you head out so that you don't arrive starving.
- ■ Make a beeline for the healthiest nibbles: olives, pickled onions, prawns, thinly sliced ham, sushi or crudités with hummus or salsa.
- ■ Plan your alcohol strategy: avoid it altogether by offering to be the Designated Driver; pour yourself an alcoholic and a large non-alcoholic, low-cal drink simultaneously and don't fetch refills until you've finished both drinks; use the alcohol in your daily Snacks/Extras allocation and/or go for low-cal options, such as a measure of spirits with a low-cal mixer.

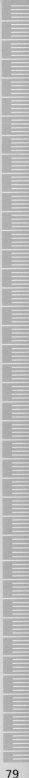

WHAT LISA LEARNED

I don't believe in having 'diet' foods in my house, as they send out a signal to me that I'm on diet, which I'm not! I never lost weight when I lived on diet foods and low-fat biscuits, so now I avoid them completely. Interestingly, research[25] shows that when people opt for low-fat/diet foods, they eat more of them as they think they're low-calorie/calorie-free, and that's certainly something I've found to be true for me and my patients. Yes, I eat low-fat yogurts (but I avoid ones with the sweetener aspartame, as I don't like putting weird chemicals into my body) and only use skimmed milk because that's an easy way to reduce my calorie intake, but I don't have anything in my home that screams 'diet' at me every time I open a cupboard.

The five best investments I've made have been a non-stick frying pan (so I use less oil when cooking), an electric steamer with a timer (so I can cook my veggies while having a shower after my evening run without fearing that they'll burn or go mushy), a hand-held blender (so I can whip up slimming soups in seconds), loads of plastic clip-lock food-storage containers (so I can carry muesli and nuts around with me and freeze meals I've cooked in quantity) and beautiful square dinner plates that turn every meal into a special, life-affirming occasion.

The food I adore the most is… fish and chips! So how have I remained on first-name terms with the super-friendly staff of Ossies Fish & Chips up the road (Hi there, Nazmi, Hasim and baby Sultannur) and still managed to stay slim? Firstly, I always order a really large portion of fish and two portions of mushy peas (and pinch a few chips off my husband's plate – you can always ask for a quarter portion, if you like). Secondly, I only ever eat a tiny amount of the batter. Finally, I only go there once a month now (my former record was four times in one week!).

Nothing is more off-putting than opening your fridge and being faced with a mountain of composting vegetables, so I wash and freeze fresh veggies I've bought if I think they might go off before I can cook them (I've found there's no need for fiddly blanching) and add them to stews and soups when I need them. And when I've bought growing herbs and don't think I'll use them up in time, I cut off the leaves and pop them in the freezer in airtight bags for later, too.

As a child, I was crazy about buffets. Now I'm older and wiser I know they can pose a serious threat to my figure, so on a visit to Vegas (the spiritual heartland of all-you-can-eat) I perfected my buffet survival skills. First I scope out what's on offer and decide whether I'm going to have dessert (which will influence how many high-calorie mouthfuls I'll allow for my main course). Then I have a plate of salad or soup. I always have a little of whatever high-calorie foods I fancy, but I make sure that at least half my plate is full of tasty veggies or salad. And I seldom go back for seconds. If I do, I allow myself just one or two tablespoons of whatever delighted me first time round, and leave it at that. Simple.

> ## 66 If you eat out a lot, decide beforehand whether you're going to have bread, wine or dessert – never all three 99

Ever envy your slim friends who seem to be effortlessly slim while you gain weight just licking a postage stamp? Don't! What I've noticed over the years is that their 'natural' slimness isn't as mysterious as I once thought: yes, they don't endlessly obsess about their weight, but they're constantly making tiny good decisions throughout the day that help them to maintain their figure. Once I became aware of this, I turned into a Slimming Spy and began to adopt a few of their tactics myself. My colleague Tara (a Goal Group member), for example, seldom said 'No' to the tempting goodies passed round the office, but then she also never failed to refuse second helpings of them either. And my neighbour Dragana taught me the best way to cook something that takes a bit of time, like a stew. She feels more energetic after dinner, so that's when she does all her chopping. She then pops the stew in the oven, settles down to watch a movie for two hours and then turns off the oven before bed. The next day, she can look forward to a healthy meal that just needs

reheating (oh, and she always cooks double portions so there's one for the freezer). Celebrities can also provide fab slimming tips if you choose ones that don't live on caffeine and nicotine. One, for example, taught me that whenever she went out to a red-carpet do, she'd decide beforehand whether she'd have either bread, wine or dessert – never all three.

I confess to being hopelessly and utterly devoted to tea and use it to stave off boredom, the cold - and hunger pangs! By drinking decaf and herbal teas I've found I can have as much as I want without the caffeine side effects. To keep things interesting, I have a cute canister of different teas on my desk and I pick one out at random each time I fancy a heart-warming cuppa (I call it playing the Tea Lottery).

One of the greatest revelations I've had is that you can cook a lot of things from frozen. When I got home late at night I used to look in vain for something to eat, realise I'd forgotten to defrost anything and promptly dial for a takeaway. Now that my freezer is jam-packed with frozen prawns, fish and mussels, chopped-up chicken and meat and veggies, I know I can always cook a healthy dinner at a dash. I just grab a handful of frozen protein-rich food, two handfuls of frozen veg, a can of chopped tomatoes and, hey presto, I've got an utterly delicious dish in less time than it takes for the takeaway delivery man to hop on his motorbike.

CHOOSING YOUR CHANGES

Now you know exactly what to do to whittle your waist, boost your wellbeing and continue adoring yourself slim. However, from my work with patients over the years, I realise that it can feel overwhelming to have to make all these changes all at once. Lyndel agrees. This is why I've devised an Adoption Certificate that will enable you either to adopt the plan wholesale, as I did, or just choose a few elements from it to start with and build from there. Once those changes have become a habit (some already may be!), you can add some more if you want to, until you've revamped your lifestyle in a way that works for you. If you're going for the softly, softly approach, I suggest deciding on just two or three things that you think will be really easy, and then diarising them or putting them on Post-its around your home as a reminder.

SET THE SCENE FOR SUCCESS

Before you put your changes into action, ask yourself the following questions:
■ What needs to be in place? For example, if you've chosen to start having three regular meals a day, how will you make that happen? What foods do you need to buy? What kitchen equipment (such as a steamer or airtight containers) do you need? What times is it practical to eat?
■ What might make it difficult for you to implement each change?
■ How might those difficulties be overcome?
   Now's also the time to continue filling in your *Adore Yourself Slim* Travel Journal (see page 148) and the compliments you receive (see page 147). Set aside time to do this every day and you'll have a permanent record of everything you've done to achieve your goals that you'll look back on with pride once you've reached your Destination Dream Weight.

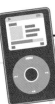

HYPNOTISE YOURSELF SLIM: TRACK 2

Having used your conscious mind to decide on the life-affirming changes you're going to make, you'll now use your unconscious mind to unlearn unhelpful habits and learn new, more positive ones. You're now ready to listen to Track 2 (Eat Yourself Slim) on your hypnosis CD. Play this 16-minute track first thing in the morning and last thing at night (there's no need to wake up afterwards – you can just allow yourself to drift off to sleep). If you find it hard to fit an extra 16 minutes into your morning routine, listen to this track while commuting (remember, however, that you shouldn't play it when driving, as it could make you lose concentration or go into a hypnotic state at the wheel). If you forget to do it first thing (or run out of time), then skip the introduction and countdown, and simply listen to the suggestions while you have breakfast or walk to work.

The time you spend listening to this track each day will make the most amazing difference to the way you feel about healthy eating (think of it as your Secret Slimming Tool). It'll help you lose the taste for toxic 'treats' and energy-sapping junk calories, and develop a new desire to eat the foods that nurture and nourish both your body and soul.

ADOPTION CERTIFICATE

This is to certify that I,

_____

solemnly declare that I will adopt the following lifestyle changes, starting on the dates specified (but accept that there'll be ups and downs along the way, so I vow not to be too hard on myself!), as I embark on the journey of a lifetime.

	Date of commitment	Still doing it 1 week later	Still doing it 2 weeks later	Still doing it 3 weeks later	Still doing it 4 weeks later	Still doing it 2 months later	Still doing it 3 months later
Putting myself first							
Asking: 'What do I *really* need right now' when I feel hungry							
Eating three meals and two snacks a day							
Eating at least five portions of fruit and veg a day							
Drinking plenty of fluids							
Getting enough rest and sleep							
Listening to my hypnosis CD							
Shopping on a set day each week							
Sitting down when eating (even for snacks!), eating slowly and mindfully and stopping when I'm full							
Watching my portion sizes							
Limiting my alcohol intake							
Weighing and measuring myself regularly							
Rewarding myself regularly							
Writing down my compliments							
Filling in my *Adore Yourself Slim* Travel Journal							
Becoming more active (see Chapter 5 for more on this)							

THE RECIPES THAT'LL HELP YOU ADORE YOURSELF SLIM

I don't like slimming books with lots of recipes, as they just intimidate me and make me feel that I'm not the domestic goddess I should be. Most of the food I cook is what my Dad calls 'chuck-it-in cuisine' – I simply make things in a tearing hurry that I think will taste good using the ingredients listed on pages 69–71. However, I couldn't resist including a selection of my favourite recipes, which have delighted my taste buds (and, I hope, those of my dinner guests!) for several years now. All can be whipped up in under 30 minutes so they fit into a hectic lifestyle. As I dislike recipes with ingredients lists a mile long, I've chosen ones that contain mainly storecupboard ingredients – with a few fresh or frozen ingredients thrown in.

I hope you adore my recipes as much as I do, but if you don't, don't despair – adapt these to suit your taste (never let a missing ingredient deter you from attempting a recipe – simply substitute a similar ingredient), trawl the internet for healthy alternatives or badger your friends for suggestions. It's a great idea to buy a file and label it DINNER WHEN I'M DESPERATE and then add any quick-and-easy recipes you come across. The hour before dinner is the time most of us are tempted to cave in and snack on cheese or crisps as we wait for our meal to cook, so knowing that you have simple make-in-minutes recipes you can rustle up is vital to slimming success. Don't forget to make double

> **66 Knowing you have simple make-in-minutes dinner recipes you can rustle up is vital to slimming success 99**

quantities where you can and freeze them, if appropriate, for super-speedy weeknight dinners.

I've indicated the number of servings of each food group that each recipe contains, but do bear in mind that this doesn't include the serving suggestions (or veggies you'll be having), which should be added separately. You'll notice that most of the recipes are low-carb rather than moderate-carb – that's because I've usually used up my Nutritious Carbohydrates allocation by dinnertime! If you haven't, by all means add a serving (or two) of wholewheat pasta, bread, rice or potatoes (this is also what Lyndel suggests if you're cooking for family members who don't need to lose weight – see page 65).

All the recipes serve four, so they're family friendly, but you can double, halve or quarter the quantities if you need to. Also, I've suggested my favourite veggies to go with them, but please feel free to choose at least two servings per meal of your own. Happy cooking!

VEGETARIAN

Vegetables are good sources of many vitamins and minerals, yet most of us don't eat nearly enough of them. This is a bit baffling considering that they taste utterly delicious (and the UK Food Standards Agency says there's evidence to suggest that eating lots of fruit and veg means you're less likely to develop chronic diseases such as coronary heart disease and some cancers). Veg are also very low in fat and most are very low-cal, too, so pile your plate with them. I've included some of my all-time favourite veggie recipes here – all are tasty enough to be served at dinner parties and, even if you're a committed carnivore, won't make you feel that you're missing out on meat if you have them as a main meal.

VERY LOW CAL

▶ TRIUMPH SOUP
¼ Dairy; 1 Fat serving per portion

I've been making this inexpensive but luxe-tasting soup for over 15 years and it never fails to impress dinner-party guests, even though I've adapted it to contain only a smidgen of oil, unlike the butter-heavy original. The name comes from my reaction when I first made it as a very unconfident cook. I lifted the lid of the pot and, on smelling the fragrant combination of carrot and caraway, called out to my husband excitedly: 'I think this is going to be a triumph!' It makes a great Sanity Saver (see page 72).

- 1 large onion, sliced
- 4 tsp extra-virgin olive oil
- 500g (1lb 2oz) carrots, peeled and sliced
- 2 tsp caraway seeds
- 1 bouquet garni sachet
- 2 garlic cloves, crushed
- salt and freshly ground black pepper
- 1 litre (1¾ pints) chicken stock
- 200ml (7fl oz) semi-skimmed milk

1 Sweat the onion with the oil in a large covered pan over a very low heat until soft (don't allow the onion to brown), stirring occasionally. Except for the stock and milk, add all the other ingredients, along with some salt and pepper, and continue to cook over a very low heat for 5 minutes, stirring occasionally.

2 Add the stock and allow to simmer, partly covered, until the carrots are tender. Remove the bouquet garni and, using a hand-held blender, blend the soup until smooth. Then add the milk and heat until the soup is piping hot. Divide between 4 soup bowls, garnish with some ground black pepper and serve with a slice of toasted rye bread.

▶ BUTTERNUT TAGINE
1½ Protein; 1 Dairy; 1 Fat serving per portion

- 4 tsp extra-virgin olive oil
- 2 onions, finely chopped
- 4 garlic cloves, crushed
- 2 tsp ground turmeric
- 1 tsp cumin seeds
- 1 tsp ground cinnamon
- ½ tsp cayenne pepper
- ½ tsp freshly ground black pepper
- 1 tbsp honey
- 1 large butternut squash, peeled, deseeded and cut into small chunks
- 2 x 400g (14oz) cans chickpeas, rinsed and drained
- handful of fresh parsley, chopped
- 4 tbsp natural yogurt (per person)
- lemon wedges

1 Heat the oil in a large saucepan, add the onions and garlic and gently sauté until soft.
2 Add the spices, honey and butternut squash. Pour in just enough water to cover the base of the saucepan and cover with a lid. Cook gently for 15 minutes.
3 Add the chickpeas and a little extra water if needed. Cover with the lid and cook gently until the butternut is soft. Scatter with the parsley and serve with the yogurt and lemon wedges.

▶ ORIENTAL TOFU SALAD
½ Snack/Extra (if adding peanuts); 1 Protein; 1 Fat serving per portion

- 4 tsp toasted sesame oil
- 2 tsp sweet chilli sauce
- ½ tsp grated fresh root ginger
- 1 garlic clove, crushed
- 3 tsp soy sauce
- salt, to taste
- 400g (14oz) firm tofu, cut into bite-sized cubes
- 1 small onion, quartered and finely sliced
- 200g (7oz) mange tout, cut into long strips
- 200g (7oz) red cabbage, finely shredded
- 4 carrots, peeled and cut into strips
- 2 small handfuls of peanuts (optional)

1 Place the oil, chilli sauce, ginger, garlic, soy sauce, salt and tofu in a bowl, mix well, then cover and allow to marinate while you make the salad.
2 Prepare the remaining salad ingredients and then add them to the tofu and toss well. Sprinkle with the peanuts, if using, and serve. This salad can be made in advance and improves by being left to stand for a few hours so that the flavours permeate the tofu.

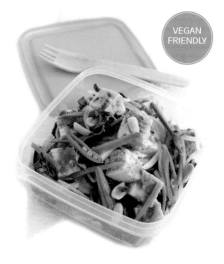

VEGAN FRIENDLY

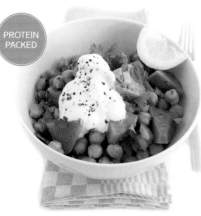

PROTEIN PACKED

ROASTED FETA VEGETABLES

1 Nutritious Carbohydrates; 2 Dairy; 1½ Fat servings per portion

- 4 courgettes, trimmed and sliced
- 1 aubergine, trimmed and sliced
- 4 medium or 2 large sweet potatoes, unpeeled, scrubbed and thinly sliced
- 2 red or green peppers, deseeded and sliced
- 2 large red onions, sliced
- 4 tomatoes, sliced
- 4 garlic cloves, thickly sliced
- 1 tbsp balsamic vinegar
- 2 tbsp extra-virgin olive oil
- salt and freshly ground black pepper
- 224g (8oz) feta or halloumi cheese, diced
- 24 olives

1 Preheat the oven to 200°C/400°F/gas mark 6. Place all the vegetables in a large baking dish, along with the garlic, vinegar, oil and seasoning, and toss well. Place the dish in the oven and roast for 40 minutes.

2 Add the cheese and olives and roast for a further 10 minutes or until the vegetables are cooked through, then serve.

ISCHIA PASTA

2 Nutritious Carbohydrates; 1 Dairy; 1 Fat serving per portion

- 224g (8oz) dried wholewheat spaghetti
- 4 tsp extra-virgin olive oil
- 1½ bunches spring onions, sliced
- 6 garlic cloves, finely sliced
- 3 x 275g (9½oz) punnets cherry tomatoes, halved
- 4 tsp dried thyme
- 6 tsp dried chives
- 2 big squeezes of tomato purée or to taste
- salt, to taste
- handful of fresh basil leaves, shredded
- 112g (4oz) Parmesan cheese, grated

1 Cook the spaghetti according to the packet instructions. Meanwhile, add the oil to a pan, heat over a high heat and then fry the spring onions and garlic for 5 minutes, stirring often.

2 Add the tomato halves to the pan and cook over a high heat for 1 minute, then reduce the heat, add the herbs, tomato purée and salt to taste and cook for 3–4 minutes, stirring.

3 Add 2 tbsp of hot water to the pan and squash a few of the tomatoes. Add the pasta to the sauce and stir over a low heat. Add the basil and stir in. Sprinkle with the Parmesan and serve with a large side salad.

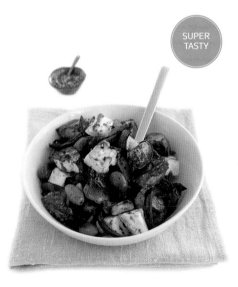

SUPER TASTY

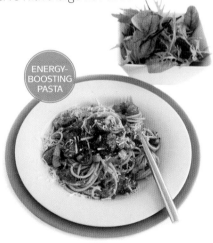

ENERGY-BOOSTING PASTA

CHICKEN

Chicken is an excellent source of filling protein. Remember, however, that chicken skin is high in unwanted fat and should be removed before eating. Chicken is amazingly versatile – I often just griddle or roast a chicken breast and serve it spread with a teaspoonful of low-sugar jam or lime pickle. It's also very easy to throw together a chicken stew: just brown some chopped chicken breast, add a few handfuls of veggies, cover in stock and simmer until tender.

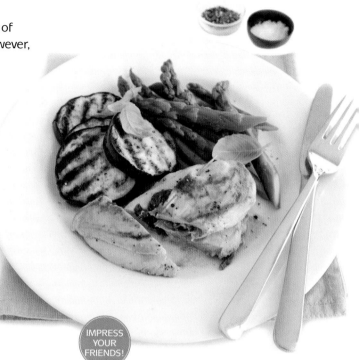

IMPRESS YOUR FRIENDS!

▶ CHICKEN SALTIMBOCCA

2½ Protein; 1 Fat serving per portion

- 4 x 150g (5½oz) skinless chicken breasts
- 16 large basil leaves, plus extra to garnish
- 4 slices of prosciutto or Parma ham
- ½ x 225g (8oz) bag spinach, washed, wilted and excess water removed
- 4 tsp extra-virgin olive oil
- 200ml (7fl oz) chicken stock
- 2 tbsp lemon juice

1 Cut all four of the chicken breasts in half horizontally, leaving one side attached. Open them out like a book and lay 4 basil leaves inside each of them, followed by a slice of prosciutto and a quarter of the spinach. Close and 'sew up' each breast with a couple of wooden cocktail sticks or a wooden skewer.

2 Heat the olive oil in a large, non-stick frying pan and add the chicken breasts. Cook for 3 minutes until golden, then turn over and cook for a further 2 minutes. Add the chicken stock and lemon juice and simmer until the chicken is cooked through. Remove the chicken breasts and keep warm by wrapping them in foil while boiling the pan juices so that they reduce into a sauce.

3 Pour the sauce over the chicken, garnish with some extra basil leaves and serve with griddled aubergine slices and steamed asparagus spears. To make the aubergine, simply brush some aubergine slices with olive oil and cook until soft in a very hot griddle pan.

AUNTY JOANIE'S CHICKEN

2 Protein; ½ Fat serving per portion

My fabulously theatrical Aunt Joan introduced us to this super-simple, heart-warming dish at a family get-together. When pressed for the recipe and its name, she simply replied: 'It's called chicken! It's just the way I always cook chicken.' Hence it's now called Aunty Joanie's chicken! Bones add flavour, so use chicken on the bone where possible.

- 600g (1lb 5oz) skinless chicken thighs or breasts
- 10 cloves
- 2 large onions, chopped
- 7 tbsp malt vinegar
- 2 tsp extra-virgin olive oil

1 Place the chicken in a large pot and cover with water. Add all the other ingredients and simmer, uncovered, until the liquid has been reduced by at least half and the chicken is thoroughly cooked. The longer you cook this dish, the more melt-in-the-mouth the chicken becomes. You can freeze any leftover liquid and use it as a stock for chicken soup or stew.
2 Serve with steamed Savoy cabbage and mashed swede.

MARMALADE CHICKEN

1 Snack/Extra; 2 Protein; 1 Fat serving per portion

- 2 teacups or 500ml (18fl oz) chicken stock
- 4 tbsp red wine vinegar
- 4 tbsp orange marmalade
- 2 tsp Dijon mustard
- 2 tsp cornflour
- salt and freshly ground black pepper
- 4 tsp extra-virgin olive oil
- 600g (1lb 5oz) skinless chicken breasts, cut into strips
- 6 small onions, finely chopped
- 4 spring onions, diagonally sliced
- 1 tsp freshly grated orange zest

1 Whisk the stock, vinegar, marmalade, mustard and cornflour together in a bowl.
2 Season the chicken with salt and pepper. Heat 3 tsp of the oil in a non-stick saucepan over a medium-high heat. Add the chicken, cook until golden, then remove and set aside.
3 Add the remaining 1 tsp oil to the pan, along with the onions and spring onions, and cook, stirring often, until beginning to brown. Whisk the stock mixture and add it to the pan. Bring to a simmer, scraping up any browned bits. Reduce the heat and cook until the sauce has thickened. Add the chicken and cook until it's heated through. Stir in the orange zest and serve with steamed broccoli and courgettes.

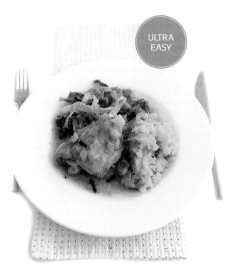

ULTRA EASY

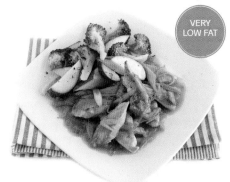

VERY LOW FAT

FISH

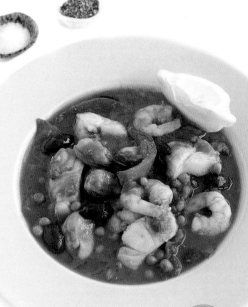

Fish ranks second highest on the satiety index (a measure of how satisfied you feel after eating a meal) developed by researchers at the University of Sydney[26]. It's rich in protein and has a low energy density (meaning fewer calories per mouthful), so it's great for naturally switching off hunger signals to help you stop eating when you're full.

The UK Food Standards Agency recommends that we eat at least two portions of fish a week, including one of oily fish. Oily fish also provides plenty of heart-healthy, metabolism-, mood- and immune-system-supporting omega-3 fats. Remember that while fresh tuna is an oily fish, and so is high in omega-3s, it's cooked before it's canned, which reduces these fatty acids to levels similar to white fish, so, in the nutrition stakes, canned tuna doesn't count as oily fish. As oily fish can contain small amounts of pollutants, pregnant or breastfeeding women are advised to have no more than two 140g (5oz) servings a week (the same applies if there's a chance that you could become pregnant). Women who will not be having children in the future, and men and boys, can have up to four portions a week. To find out which types of fish come from sustainable sources, visit www.fishonline.org.

CHUCK-IT-IN CUISINE!

▶ NO-RICE PAELLA

2 Protein; 1 Nutritious Carbohydrates; ½ Fat serving per portion

- 2 tsp extra-virgin olive oil
- 300g (10½oz) frozen pollock fillets, or other white fish from sustainable sources
- 2 x 400g (14oz) cans chopped tomatoes
- good squeeze of tomato purée (optional)
- 4 garlic cloves, peeled and crushed
- 4 red peppers, deseeded and sliced
- 24 Kalamata olives, stoned and halved
- 1 teacup or 125g (4½oz) frozen peas
- 4 tbsp capers (optional)
- freshly ground black pepper
- 200g (7oz) frozen cooked shelled mussels
- 200g (7oz) frozen cooked peeled prawns
- lemon wedges, to garnish

1 Heat the oil in a large pan and add the frozen pollock fillets, cooking gently until the fish is defrosted. Add all the other ingredients, except the seafood and lemon wedges, and allow to simmer until the peppers are soft and the fish can be broken into bite-sized pieces.

2 Add the mussels and prawns and simmer for a further 5 minutes. Serve, garnished with the lemon wedges.

SALMON & ORANGE SAUCE

**1 Snack/Extra; 1 Fruit; 2 Protein;
1 Fat serving per portion**

This is a fantastic way to turn a simple piece of grilled salmon into a restaurant-style meal. An easy variation is to add one or more of the following: 2 tbsp soy sauce, 1 tbsp ground ginger, 2 crushed garlic cloves and 1 tsp dried rosemary.

- juice of 4 oranges
- zest of 2 oranges
- 4 tbsp honey
- 4 tsp extra-virgin olive oil
- 4 x 150g (5½oz) salmon fillets, rinsed

1 Add the orange juice, orange zest and honey to a saucepan and simmer until the liquid has reduced enough to form a sauce.

2 Heat the oil in a non-stick frying pan and fry the salmon over a medium heat until it's cooked, turning once.

3 Pour the orange and honey sauce over the salmon and serve with wilted spinach and steamed carrots.

MOOD BOOSTING

SALMON & STEM GINGER

**½ Fruit; 2 Protein; 2 Fat servings
per portion**

This recipe is inspired by Rick Stein's fabulous Salmon en Croute with Currants and Ginger that drew gasps of admiration when I cooked it for a dinner party. This version is no less mouthwatering, but reduces the unfeasible amounts of butter and eliminates the sinful pastry. Whoever said 'diet' food had to be dull?

- 4 tsp extra-virgin olive oil
- 4 x 150g (5½oz) salmon fillets, rinsed
- 4 tsp butter
- 2 heaped tbsp currants or raisins
- 8 pieces of stem ginger in syrup, drained and finely sliced
- salt and freshly ground black pepper

1 Heat the oil in a non-stick frying pan and fry the salmon over a medium heat until it's cooked, turning once.

2 In a small saucepan, gently heat the butter, then add the currants and stem ginger. Season well and heat through.

3 Pour the ginger and currant butter over the salmon and serve with a selection of steamed vegetables, such as mange tout and leeks.

DINNER-PARTY FARE

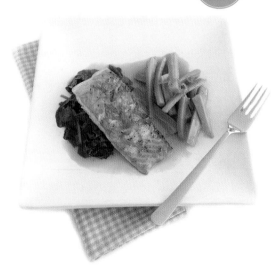

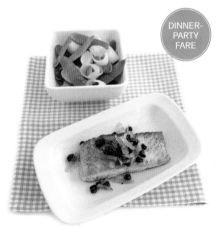

PORK AND BEEF

Meat is a good source of protein, vitamins and minerals, such as iron (which helps make red blood cells, needed to carry oxygen around your body) and immunity-boosting zinc. It's also one of the main sources of vitamin B12, which helps to keep our nervous system healthy and also helps to make red blood cells. Some types of meat are high in fat, particularly saturated fat, which can raise cholesterol levels and so increase your chances of developing heart disease. Hence, when buying pork or beef, look for the leanest cuts (choose the leanest mince, too), and remove any visible fat before cooking. It's best to limit red meat to three or four times a week to allow for fish, vegetable dishes and chicken to be included in your diet and so keep it balanced.

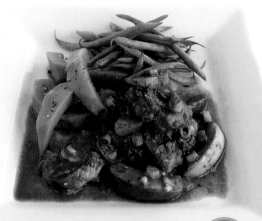

COMFORT FOOD

▶ PORK & CIDER SAUCE
½ **Snack/Extra**; ½ **Fruit**; 2 **Protein**; 1½ **Fat servings per portion**

- 3 tbsp plain flour
- salt and freshly ground black pepper
- 600g (1lb 5oz) pork tenderloin fillet, cut into 1cm (½in) thick slices
- 2 tbsp butter
- 1 red onion, halved and finely sliced
- 2 red apples, cored and sliced
- 8 spring onions, trimmed and sliced
- 150ml (5fl oz) dry cider
- 1 tbsp honey
- 1 tsp tomato purée
- 1 tbsp semi-skimmed milk

1 Place the flour, salt and pepper in a sandwich bag, add the pork slices in small batches and toss until the pork is thoroughly coated.
2 Melt the butter in a large, non-stick frying pan over a medium heat. When it stops foaming, add the pork and fry over a medium heat until well browned. Remove from the pan and set aside.
3 Add the red onion to the pan and soften over a very low heat. Turn the heat up to medium, then add the apple slices and cook, stirring frequently, until the apple is soft and browned. Add the spring onions, cider, honey and tomato purée and bring rapidly to the boil, stirring all the time. Add the milk, then season to taste with salt and pepper.
4 Add the pork to the sauce and heat until piping hot, stirring frequently. Serve with steamed green beans and butternut squash.

PARMA HAM & FIG SALAD

**½ Fruit; 2 Protein; 1 Fat serving
per portion**

During the summer months, I have a variation of this utterly delicious (and surprisingly filling) salad for lunch virtually every day. Peppadews come from my home country of South Africa and are a cross between a chilli and red pepper, so they've got a bit of bite but can be eaten whole. They come in bottles, and many of the large supermarkets stock them.

- 2 x 100g (3½oz) bags pre-prepared spinach, watercress and rocket salad
- 1 x 275g (9½oz) punnet baby tomatoes, halved
- 2 yellow peppers, deseeded and cut into rings
- 12 Peppadews, cut into quarters
- 1 onion, sliced into rings
- 16 slices of Parma ham
- 4 fresh or dried figs, cut into quarters
- balsamic vinegar, for drizzling
- 4 tsp extra-virgin olive oil

1 Arrange the salad ingredients on 4 plates, then top each serving with an equal quantity of the Parma ham slices and fig quarters.

2 Drizzle a little balsamic vinegar and 1 tsp oil over each salad and serve immediately.

HEALTHY BURGERS

**2 Protein; ½ Dairy; 1 Fat serving
per portion**

- 500g (1lb 2oz) lean mince (beef, lamb, turkey or Quorn)
- 2 eggs, beaten
- 2 small onions, chopped
- 4 garlic cloves, crushed
- 85g (3oz) watercress, finely chopped
- salt and freshly ground black pepper
- 5 tsp wholegrain mustard or curry paste
- 2 red peppers, deseeded and cut into rings
- 2 large courgettes, trimmed and sliced
- 4 tsp extra-virgin olive oil
- 8 tbsp 0% fat natural Greek yogurt
- 4 tbsp chopped fresh coriander

1 Mix together the mince, egg, onion, half the garlic, watercress, seasoning and mustard in a large bowl. Divide the mixture into 12, then shape each piece into a small, thin patty.

2 Place the pepper rings, courgette slices and oil in a bowl and toss well.

3 Make the yogurt sauce by mixing the yogurt, the remaining garlic and coriander together, then season to taste with salt and pepper.

4 Cook the burgers and vegetables under a hot grill or on a barbecue until they're cooked through. Serve with a mini wholemeal pita bread, the sauce and a green salad if you wish.

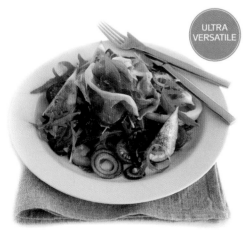

ULTRA VERSATILE

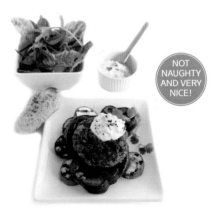

NOT NAUGHTY AND VERY NICE!

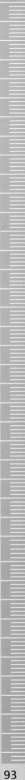

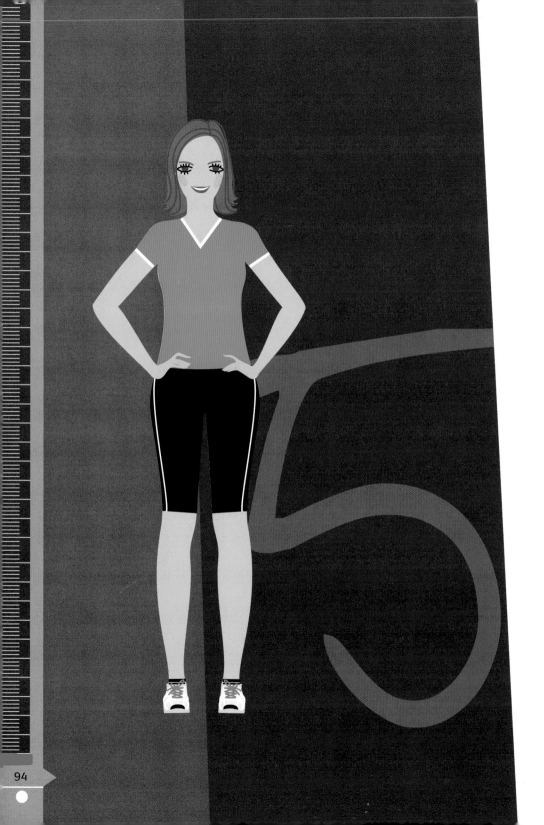

Chapter 5

EXERCISE
yourself
SLIM

Now that you know what the *Adore Yourself Slim* Eating Plan involves, it's time to turn your attention to the oft-dreaded 'e' word. Yes, exercise. Without it, you'll still lose weight if you follow the eating plan, but you'll do so more slowly, less healthily and – hence – the hard way. In other words, you'll be taking the long way round to Destination Dream Weight. And, of course, you won't look as foxy in your slimmer body if it's flabby rather than firm. Read on to discover how to get fitter in the shortest possible time – and have loads of fun while you're at it!

EXERCISE: THE SHORT CUT TO SLIM

My patients often ask me whether they have to exercise as well as eat more healthily to lose weight. After all, it seems a lot easier to step away from that tempting doughnut than it is to get hot and sweaty on a regular basis. Well, I think these statistics speak for themselves: according to 2005 data[1] from The National Weight Control Registry, an American organisation with over 4,000 members who lost at least 30lb (13.6kg) and kept it off for at least a year, a significant 89% of their members successfully lost and maintained their lower weight using diet and physical activity. This indicates that exercise is an integral part of successful fat loss, which is why I felt that it was so essential to include it in this book. Performing the type of exercise you'll be reading about in this chapter really turbocharged my own weight loss, and I'm convinced it'll do the same for you.

Another incredible benefit of exercise, according to a Dutch study[2], is that doing even just moderate activity (the equivalent of walking for 30 minutes a day, five days a week) can help women live one-and-a-half years longer than those who're less active, so giving you more time to do all those fab things on your Want-To-Do List (see page 54). Vigorous activity, by the way, which is defined as the equivalent of running for 30 minutes a day, five times a week, can extend your lifespan by an incredible three-and-a-half years.

To help you in this part of the programme I've enlisted the help of Sarah Maxwell and Coach Bronek (see page 102), two of the most inspiring fitness professionals I've come across in my 11 years of working in health journalism. Between them they have dozens of years worth of fitness experience – they've done the training, they've read the research and they've exhaustively evaluated every exercise, so you don't have to! Sarah's Sneaky Workout will show you cunning ways to slip exercise into your everyday life (so you won't even notice you're doing it!), while the two no-nonsense, fat-blasting routines devised by Coach Bronek (Six Weeks To Slim and Six Weeks To Super-Fit) are designed to help you get the most out of every nanosecond you spend exercising.

MEET SARAH MAXWELL

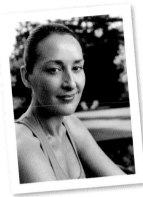

Personal trainer and lifestyle consultant Sarah Maxwell numbers *Strictly Come Dancing* stars among her star-studded client list. Whereas many personal trainers are fanatical about fitness and somehow can't comprehend that anyone could possibly prefer an evening cocooned cosily on the sofa with a pizza to a night of pumping iron at the gym, Sarah is far more realistic. 'I know that many of my clients think exercise is a pain and a drag,' she says, 'but they know it makes them look good and, more importantly, feel good, so that's why they do it. I can't force them to love working out, but my job is to make it as fun as possible – and, more importantly, to help them find ways to fit it into their manic filming or performance schedules.'

'Time is the world's most precious commodity,' says Sarah. 'In fact, it's so valuable I sometimes think it should be listed on the Stock Exchange! That's why I tell my time-poor clients to sneak exercise into each and every tiny pocket of spare time they have during the day. What many people don't realise is that doing several short bouts of exercise is almost as effective as doing a 40-minute workout.' So if you're new to exercise, or aren't yet sure how you're going to manage to fit it into your life, follow Sarah's Sneaky Workout, overleaf.

▶ FINDING THE TIME TO TRAIN

Time is often cited as the main reason most of us don't exercise. As we hurtle through life at a million miles per hour, it's hard enough to find the time to floss our teeth, let alone have time to work out. And yet time is the one thing every person on this planet has exactly the same amount of. Monk or millionaire, old or young, each and every one of us has been given the same 24 hours every day, and it's what we do with those 24 hours that counts.

If you've decided to do Sarah's Sneaky Workout, you need to mentally scour your daily schedule for any pockets of 'dead' time or habitual activities that could be put to good use for exercise (or that you can use as triggers to remind you to exercise). Not everyone commutes, or works at a desk, so just tick the boxes that apply to your lifestyle and then turn the page for Sarah's top ten double-duty, super-effective training tactics. Remember, Sarah's suggestions are simply a guide – you can mix and match exercises and time slots as much as you like.

❑ Going to the loo   ❑ Listening to music
❑ Housework   ❑ Going food shopping
❑ Gardening   ❑ Using escalators
❑ Commuting   or stairs
❑ Sitting at a desk   ❑ Playing with your kids
❑ Boiling a kettle   ❑ Running a bath
❑ Watching TV   ❑ Talking on the phone

❑ (Add your own)

❑ (Add your own)

❑ (Add your own)

MAKE THE MOST OF EVERY MINUTE

To lose weight and keep it off, you need to eat less and up the amount of calories you burn each day by getting off the bus one stop earlier… taking the stairs instead of the lift… yada, yada, yawn!

How many times have you heard this advice? And how many times have you heeded it? Be honest! The irony is, it really is million-dollar, 100%-success-guaranteed, 24-carat advice, which probably should be trademarked, but it just sounds too obvious and mundane to actually work. Surely the 12 calories you expend washing and cutting up vegetables won't make a difference? You're right, in themselves they won't matter

66 Being fit is sexy. Getting fit can be, too! 99

much (after all, you have to burn 3,500 calories to lose 1lb/0.5kg of fat, which is a lot of chopping), but remember that you're still burning more calories than if you'd chosen to opt for a bag of pre-cut veggies. Add that to dozens of other little unnoticed exercise opportunities and you'll soon have to acknowledge that yes, every little bit really does help. This every-little-bit counts approach is something known as 'integrated exercise' and experts are increasingly becoming aware of just how effective it is. Integrated exercise involves doing all your normal daily activities, but doing them with real enthusiasm. It means counteracting our modern obsession with labour-saving devices and using a little old-fashioned elbow grease to accomplish everyday tasks. So if you're gym-phobic or don't like exercise yet, this is the perfect place to start.

INVISIBLE EXERCISE OPPORTUNITIES

'The easiest way to do integrated exercise is to multi-task and to challenge yourself to find a fitness opportunity in every situation or place you find yourself in,' says Sarah Maxwell. 'Being fit is sexy – and getting fit can be, too! Be creative and treat it like a game where you're constantly on the lookout for tiny segments of time that you can use to do your Sneaky Workout.'

When starting out with The Sneaky Workout, aim to adopt just one or two of Sarah's suggestions at first, and when they've become a habit, add in another couple so that you continue to challenge your body. Remember to make a note of how many you do (and how often) in your *Adore Yourself Slim* Travel Journal (see page 148) so that you can track your progress.

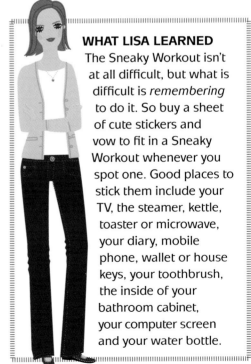

WHAT LISA LEARNED

The Sneaky Workout isn't at all difficult, but what is difficult is *remembering* to do it. So buy a sheet of cute stickers and vow to fit in a Sneaky Workout whenever you spot one. Good places to stick them include your TV, the steamer, kettle, toaster or microwave, your diary, mobile phone, wallet or house keys, your toothbrush, the inside of your bathroom cabinet, your computer screen and your water bottle.

THE SNEAKY WORKOUT

These exercises are ideal for beginners, as they're not too strenuous and you can do as many or as few as you like. Once you've got used to being more active generally, you may want to combine The Sneaky Workout with Coach Bronek's more intense workouts (see page 102) for maximum results.

1 Do walking lunges (see page 110, but omit the arm movements) while you're vacuuming. Not only will this turn your home into a haven but it'll tone your bottom and thighs and burn lots of calories, too.

2 Use your swivel chair at work to give your abs and back a Sneaky Workout. Every hour on the hour, plant your feet firmly on the floor, sit upright, pull in your abs and then twist to the right and left 20 times in a slow and controlled way.

3 Got a few minutes before going out? Put on your favourite CD and dance (perhaps drawing the curtains beforehand!). This will burn extra calories and significantly increase your bone density, making you less likely to get osteoporosis or fracture a bone in later life. What's more, the late social psychologist Professor Michael Argyle claimed that dancing gives us a greater sense of joy than anything else.

4 A watched kettle never boils, nor does a vegetable steamer, so put this time to good use by doing the plank, pliés, calf raises or side leg raises (see below), or squats (see page 105), lunges (see page 110) or beginner press-ups (see page 111).

■ **How to do... the core-strengthening plank** Rest your forearms on your kitchen worktop, place your feet as far away as you can and keep your body in a plank position (your shoulders, hips and feet should all be in the same diagonal line). Hold for 15 seconds and work up to doing 60 seconds.

■ **How to do... thigh-toning pliés** Stand with your feet hip-width apart, your abs pulled in and your hips tucked under. Take a small step out with each foot and turn your feet outwards. Place your hands on your hips or on your kitchen worktop for support. Now lower your body down slowly by bending your knees, and then return to your starting position by slowly straightening your knees. Maintain good posture by ensuring that your shoulders are back and down, your abs are pulled in and that your hips and back are aligned.

■ **How to do... calf-sculpting calf raises** Stand with your toes on a slightly raised surface so that your heels are hanging over

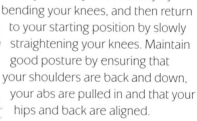

the edge (a stair tread is good). Slowly rise up on your toes, then slowly lower your heels until they're slightly below the level of your toes, and then raise your heels again.

■ **How to do... outer-thigh-shaping side leg raises** Stand side on to a table with your abs pulled in, transferring your weight onto your right leg and placing your right hand on the table to help you balance. Keep the knee of your right leg soft, not locked. Place your left hand on your hip (this is your starting position). Keep your left leg straight while raising it sideways, away from your body towards the left. When your left leg reaches a point where you feel it in your left buttock area (see the illustration on page 96), stop and hold for 1–2 seconds, then return your left leg to your starting position and repeat. Do the same number of repetitions with your right leg.

5 Cleaning your windows is a fantastic shoulder workout. Use both hands and you'll work your entire upper body. Vigorously polishing your dining-room table is another good quickie workout, as is washing your car and gardening. And when you're mopping the floor, pull in your abs and really work those arms for a full-body workout.

6 Never sit down when you're on the phone: buy a cordless phone and pace up and down, or use your talk-time to wander round the house

66 **Make like a stork and stand on one leg while chatting on the phone (or brushing your teeth) to strengthen your core stability** 99

tidying things away. Alternatively, make like a stork and stand on one leg while chatting on the phone (or brushing your teeth). This strengthens your core stability and also works your bottom and legs.

7 While you're out supermarket shopping, park as far away from the entrance as possible to build an extra few steps into your visit, and be sure to return your trolley to the store itself, rather than leaving it in the car park. You can also use your trolley to provide resistance and help flatten your tummy and promote core stability. Simply contract your pelvic-floor muscles and your abs, then use your stomach muscles, rather than your arms, to turn the trolley. This may sound a bit bonkers, but you'll soon get the hang of it. An hour of trolley pushing in this way burns an amazing 200 calories.

8 There's no need to go to the gym to use a Stairmaster – stairs are the way to get to the upper deck of the bus or to your second-floor office. Always walk up stairs two at a time, as that will tone your glutes and give you a highly desirable 'cherry butt' that will make you look fab in your jeans.

9 Make it a rule never to stand on an escalator. A trick for helping you pass the time when you're walking up an

escalator is to try to guess how many steps you'll need to get to the top, and then count each one as you go. Another way to make escalator walking enjoyable is to focus on the shoes or outfits of the people you see as you stride past them. You can even use these opportunities to glean ideas for the items you'd like to buy when you revamp your wardrobe (see page 124).

10 Buy a pedometer and wear it wherever you go. One meta-study[3] found that pedometer users increased their daily walking by an average of 2,400 steps (about a mile) – an astonishing 27% increase in activity. Aim to make your steps fast enough so that they speed up your breathing, and sneak in extra steps whenever you can: print out documents on the printer furthest from your desk and take the long route to work. For a more pricey but super-simple option, invest in a wristwatch-type GPS, which uses satellite technology to tell you exactly how fast and how far you're going – no programming required (so it's ideal for technophobes)! Record how much brisk walking you've done in your *Adore Yourself Slim* Travel Journal (see page 148) – if you've done it, write about it. The ideal number of steps for wellbeing is 10,000 per day, so see if you can work your way up to doing that…

WHAT LISA DID

Inspired by Sarah's 'anytime, anywhere' approach, I set about seeing how I could sneak exercise into my day. Here's how I did it…

■ While still working as a journalist, I'd already been using part of my evening commute to fit in a 32-minute run. But then I took the decision to walk a mile to my local station with my neighbour Theresa every morning, too, instead of getting the tram. It meant getting up ten minutes earlier each day, but the payback was sneaking in an amazing extra 100 minutes of walking a week.
■ I use tea breaks as a reminder to exercise and do either ten lunges or squats every time I switch on the kettle. It only takes about 30 seconds and I find the exercise clears my head, making me feel more alert and energised. I was surprised to learn that squats are actually easier when done in wedged heels!
■ I bought a Swiss ball and started sitting on it while at my desk to improve my posture and strengthen my core muscles. At first I got the most awful backache as my back muscles were so weak, so I started out doing just 20 minutes at a time and worked up from there. The secret is to wedge your heels under the ball so that your back is more upright.
■ I used to utterly detest walking up stairs, but now I play a live Billy Joel soundtrack on my iPod whenever I'm about to tackle a Tube escalator or stairwell. I pretend the enthusiastic applause is meant for me and, before I know it, I find I'm at the top.

FAST FORWARD TO FIT

If you're ready for a bigger commitment, and even more astonishing results, then combine The Sneaky Workout with the routines devised by my second expert, Coach Bronek, the trainer I turned to in desperation when, after going to the gym three times a week for three years and getting nowhere (as I wasn't following a structured programme), I despaired of ever losing weight. Known for his unorthodox techniques, Coach Bronek has a Masters degree in sports science and over two decades of experience in coaching everyone from fitness-phobes (like I used to be) to Paralympic medal winners.

If you've become disillusioned with the weight-loss potential of exercise over the years, take heart: I used to be pretty disappointed by it myself! Having become a marathon runner at the age of 31, I expected my new sport to turn me into a lean, mean running machine. But, despite exercising for up to seven hours a week at times, I never lost much more than a gram or two. Yes, really. This was another reason I lost hope of ever slimming down – if going from committed couch potato to marathon runner couldn't solve my weight problem, what could? The answer was a new approach to eating – plus Coach Bronek's fantastic training routines, which are super-intense but come with a no-waffle guarantee. With his help I lost just over 2½st (16.3kg) in just two-and-a-half months, and regained my faith in exercise as a weight-loss tool.

So what was I doing wrong when I was exercising for seven hours a week? According to Coach Bronek, it was the *type* of exercise I was doing that was at fault. In one experiment[4], the diet-and-moderate-cardio group (who exercised three times a week for between 30 and 50 minutes over three months) lost a paltry *1lb (0.5kg)* more weight than the diet-only group (I bet, like me, they were livid!). But fascinatingly, the diet-and-cardio-and-resistance group lost 6.5lb (2.9kg) more than the diet-only group (because resistance exercise significantly increases your metabolic rate). So that's why Coach Bronek's going to prescribe resistance exercises for you.

TURBO-CHARGED WEIGHT LOSS

But resistance exercise isn't the only key to greater weight-loss results. 'Scientists[4,5] point out that when resistance training is combined with high-intensity cardio (rather than moderate-intensity, which is nonetheless worth doing, as it's so good for the health of your heart), there's much greater potential for weight loss, especially if you also restrict your calorie intake,' says Coach Bronek. (This would explain why the hours of super-slow running I'd been doing had had so little effect on my weight.) 'So, for example, when scientists[6] compared the fat-loss-inducing potential of high-intensity interval training (HIIT) versus moderate-intensity cardio, they found that the high-intensity group lost a staggering *nine times* more subcutaneous fat (the fat just below your skin) than the other group.' If this doesn't convince you that Coach Bronek's 'difficult but deadly' HIIT cardio sessions – which we've called Power Cardio Sessions here to make them sound less scary – are worth it, nothing will!

WELCOME TO THE EXERCISE ROUTINES

Now that you're all revved up and ready to go, you'll want to know what you'll be doing to get those rapid results I promised you. What follows are two of Coach Bronek's most effective but fast routines – Six Weeks To Slim and Six Weeks To Super-Fit – and here's what you'll be doing in each of them:

a) 20-minute resistance workouts two to three times a week.[7]

b) 15–45 minutes of moderate-intensity cardio incorporated into your daily lifestyle.

c) 15–20 minutes of high-intensity cardio (Power Cardio Sessions) two to three times a week.

According to Coach Bronek, this workout combination results in maximum weight loss, so it's a plan you can be sure will work.

a) Resistance workouts

The two resistance workouts (The Let's Get Moving! Workout and The Let's Get A Move On! Workout) are designed to give maximum results in the minimum amount of time by using your large muscle groups (such as those in your bottom and thighs), which burn more calories. Each is six weeks long, because after that your body gets used to them and needs new challenges to ensure you keep progressing. 'When starting out with The Let's Get Moving! Workout, I'm suggesting you do two 20-minute resistance sessions a week (they can easily be done in your lunch-hour or before dinner),' says Coach Bronek. 'You'll build up to the recommended three when you start doing the more advanced Let's Get A Move On! Workout later on.'

b) Moderate-intensity cardio

You'll also incorporate moderate-intensity cardio training into your everyday life so that it doesn't take up too much time. This could include a brisk walk to the train/Tube/bus station, playing with your children or rushing around the house while cleaning.

c) High-intensity cardio (Power Cardio Sessions)

The Six Weeks To Slim routine involves doing two 15-minute Power Cardio Sessions a week. Later on, in the Six Weeks To Super-Fit routine, you work up to doing three 20-minute sessions a week. The time you spend doing your Power Cardio Sessions is included as part of your allotted 15–45 minutes of moderate-intensity cardio for the day, *not additional to it,* and you can choose to incorporate your Power Cardio Sessions into a moderate-cardio session or do them at a different time of day.

> ### LISA'S TOP TIP
> When you decide to follow Coach Bronek's routines, take a look at your diary at the start of each week and schedule in your activity slots by diarising them. Prioritising working out in this way means you'll be less likely to skip workouts because you'll be fitting in your other commitments around them.

The small print Coach Bronek has taken great care in devising these routines to make them as safe as possible. However, if you're new to physical exercise, or haven't exercised for a long time, please consult your GP before undertaking any strenuous exercise programme. Aim to have at least one rest day between resistance workouts, and avoid doing your resistance workout on the same day as your Power Cardio Session.

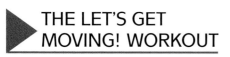

SIX WEEKS TO SLIM

TYPE OF TRAINING	WORKOUT NAME	TIME NEEDED	FREQUENCY
a) Resistance (in the form of a circuit)	The Let's Get Moving! Workout	20 minutes	Twice a week
b) Moderate-intensity cardio	'Informal' cardio in the form of walking, housework, The Sneaky Workout, etc	15–45 minutes	Daily
c) High-intensity cardio	Power Cardio Session	15 minutes	Twice a week

THE LET'S GET MOVING! WORKOUT

■ Before you start, make sure you've bought a good sports bra and a decent pair of trainers.
■ After doing your warm-up, all six exercises (which are known as a circuit) should be done in a *controlled,* continuous fashion, with the minimum amount of rest between repetitions. In the long run, aim to do all six exercises with no breaks in between.
■ Once you've finished doing your first circuit, say 'Well done, you! You're totally amazing!' to yourself several times as you rest for no longer than two minutes. Then repeat the entire circuit again. Finally, do a few of your favourite stretches (see Coach Bronek's website, www.coachbronek.com).
■ In Week 3, introduce a third circuit to your routine, having had a two-minute pep-talking rest after the second circuit. However, if you feel that you need a little more time, or find that doing two circuits is still challenging, aim to progress to doing the additional circuit and having shorter rest periods gradually.
■ If you feel you need more of a challenge, you can introduce a fourth circuit in Week 5.

■ Remember to take the time to learn the correct (and safe) way to do these exercises. If you have any doubts, ask someone at a gym to help you or hire a personal trainer for a few sessions.

THE WARM-UP

1) Walk energetically on the spot, lifting your knees as high as you can and vigorously swinging your arms for 30 seconds.
2) Jog on the spot for 30 seconds.
3) Repeat steps 1 and 2 three times, with minimal rest between them.

EXERCISE	REPETITIONS
1 Squats	8–10 repetitions
2 Split squats	6–8 repetitions on each leg
3 Modified side plank lifts	6–8 repetitions on each side
4 Side press-ups	8–10 repetitions on each side
5 Modified side leg raises	6–8 repetitions on each side
6 Rock & rolls	12–15 repetitions

1 SQUATS

'Oh noooooo! Not squats!' I hear you cry. Before you throw your hands up in despair, pause for a minute to see what Coach Bronek has to say about this exercise. 'Squats,' he says, 'are my all-time favourite exercise – if I was forced to choose just one move that gives maximum results, for either my own or my clients' training, they would be it.' So if you want a pert bottom and lithe legs, start loving those squats!

a) Stand with your feet slightly wider than hip-width apart and your toes pointing slightly outwards. Keep your arms folded in front of your chest.

b) Now bend at the hips and push your bottom out and backwards as you bend your knees, keeping your knees pushed apart, while lowering your bottom as low as you can, as if you're about to sit down on a chair (as illustrated).

c) Once you've gone as low as you can go with good technique, slowly reverse the movement and stand upright again.

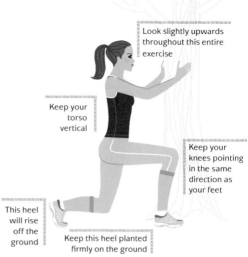

Look slightly upwards throughout this entire exercise

Keep your torso vertical

Keep your knees pointing in the same direction as your feet

This heel will rise off the ground

Keep this heel planted firmly on the ground

2 SPLIT SQUATS

Now you've realised that squats aren't as bad as you thought, it's time to do some split squats, which will help you say 'Hello, jeans! Hello, bikini!' And 'Bye, bye wobbly bottom!'

a) Stand with your feet about 1m (3ft) apart, with one foot forwards and the other behind you – this is your starting position.

b) Lower the knee of your rear leg until it nearly touches the ground (as illustrated), then return to your starting position. You can hold onto a support, such as a tree, while you do this to keep your balance. Perform the recommended number of repetitions on one leg, and then swap legs and repeat.

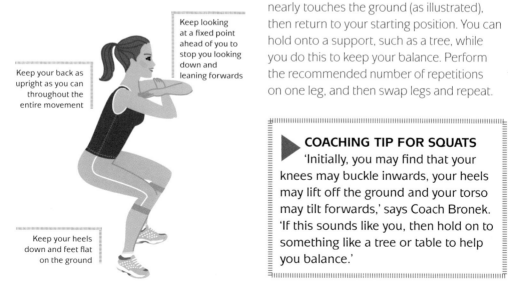

Keep your back as upright as you can throughout the entire movement

Keep looking at a fixed point ahead of you to stop you looking down and leaning forwards

Keep your heels down and feet flat on the ground

> ▶ **COACHING TIP FOR SQUATS**
> 'Initially, you may find that your knees may buckle inwards, your heels may lift off the ground and your torso may tilt forwards,' says Coach Bronek. 'If this sounds like you, then hold on to something like a tree or table to help you balance.'

3 MODIFIED SIDE PLANK LIFTS

Coach Bronek has adapted this back-, shoulder- and stomach-toning move so that it also has a fat-burning effect – genius!

a) Lie on your side with your legs bent behind you, supporting yourself on your forearm.

b) Now slowly lift your hip off the ground as high as you can (as illustrated), and then lower it to the ground in a slow and controlled way, touch the ground briefly and then raise it again. Repeat this movement for the recommended number of repetitions, then swap sides.

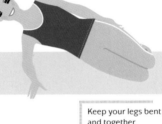
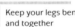

Keep your head in line with your body and look straight ahead

Keep your legs bent and together

5 MODIFIED SIDE LEG RAISES

'This will help to shape your waist and flatten your tummy,' says Coach Bronek.

a) Lie on your back with your arms stretched out to the sides. Bend your knees at right angles and lift them so that your calves are parallel to the ground.

b) Now slowly lower your knees sideways to the ground (as illustrated), then raise them back up again and slowly lower them to the other side.

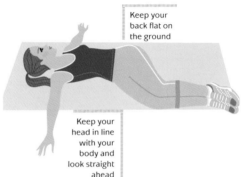

Keep your back flat on the ground

Keep your head in line with your body and look straight ahead

4 SIDE PRESS-UPS

a) Sit with your legs bent and knees pointing to the side. Place your hands on the ground to the side of you, slightly wider apart than your shoulders (this is your starting position).

b) Now bend your elbows as you lower your upper body as far as you can, so that you nearly touch your chin to the ground (as illustrated).

c) Now press your torso off the ground and return to your starting position. After completing one side, turn over and repeat the same number of press-ups on the other side.

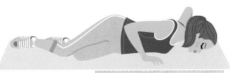

Aim to keep your nose forwards, well ahead of your hands

6 ROCK & ROLLS

And finally, a really fun-and-funky exercise that'll strengthen your abs.

a) Sit on the ground, round your back and hold your knees close to your chest using your arms – this is your starting position.

b) Now rock backwards (as illustrated), and then use the momentum you've gained to roll back forwards to your starting position.

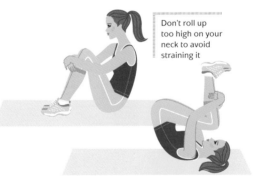

Don't roll up too high on your neck to avoid straining it

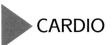

CARDIO

Your cardio consists of two components:
a) Daily moderate-intensity cardio lasting 15–45 minutes.
b) Two 15-minute high-intensity Power Cardio Sessions per week.

a) Moderate-intensity cardio

Cardio refers to any type of exercise that makes your heart beat a little faster, so you can choose whatever you like that makes you feel slightly breathless. Brisk walking, vigorous vacuuming, heavy-duty gardening or housework, using your WiiFit, playing outdoors with your kids, swimming, cycling, rowing, cross-training, skipping, trampolining, dancing and running all count. (The Sneaky Workout on page 99 has lots of other ideas on how to sneak cardio into your everyday life.) If you're new to exercise, start with brisk walks. 'I always suggest going to feed the ducks in your local park,' says Coach Bronek. 'However, don't bother to slow down to feed your ducks – the faster you whizz by them, the better! Each time you go out, time yourself and try to cover the same distance in less time. Aim to do at least 15 minutes of any of the activities mentioned above daily and gradually build up to 45 minutes.'

b) High-intensity cardio/Power Cardio Sessions

■ Once you've been walking or getting your heart pumping for up to 45 minutes regularly for two weeks, it's time to introduce 15-minute Power Cardio Sessions (otherwise known as interval training) twice a week, which means working much harder than you're used to for very short periods of time, interspersed with recovery periods where you work less hard. We'll be doing a version of the HIIT (high-intensity interval training – see page 102) that studies have shown to be an incredibly efficient fat-burner.
■ Choose an exercise you'd like to use for your training, such as cycling on a stationary bicycle, rowing on a rowing machine, using an elliptical trainer/cross-trainer or walking or running (either on a treadmill or outdoors).

▶ YOUR POWER CARDIO SESSIONS

Warm-up 5 minutes of brisk walking.
Interval 15 seconds of high-intensity exercise (if you're walking, this means power-walking; if you're running, this means sprinting or, as the T-shirt says, 'Run like you stole something!'; if you're cycling, this means pedalling like mad!).
Recovery 45 seconds of recovery (if you're walking, this means slower walking; if you're running, this means jogging; if you're cycling, this means sedate pedalling).
Repeat the Interval and Recovery sections 5 times.
Cool-down 5 minutes of brisk walking or jogging plus stretches.
TOTAL TIME 15 minutes of can't-get-any-better-fat-burning-results cardio.
■ **Week 3** Do the Power Cardio Session, above, twice a week.
■ **Week 4** Increase your Interval time to 20 seconds and decrease your Recovery time to 40 seconds.
■ **Week 5** Increase your Interval time to 25 seconds and decrease your Recovery time to 35 seconds.
■ **Week 6** Increase your Interval time to 30 seconds and decrease your Recovery time to 30 seconds.

▶ SIX WEEKS TO SUPER-FIT

TYPE OF TRAINING	WORKOUT NAME	TIME NEEDED	FREQUENCY
a) Resistance (in the form of a Superset circuit)	The Let's Get A Move On! Workout	20 minutes	Three times a week on alternate days
b) Moderate-intensity cardio	'Informal' cardio in the form of walking, housework, The Sneaky Workout, etc	15–45 minutes	Daily
c) High-intensity cardio	Power Cardio Session	16–20 minutes	Three times a week on alternate days

▶ THE LET'S GET A MOVE ON! WORKOUT

■ After your warm-up (see below right), start performing exercise 1A (Beginner burpees). When you've completed the required number of repetitions, immediately start doing exercise 1B (Star jumps). 1A and 1B together form a 'Superset' – these are designed to increase the intensity of your workout significantly and hence your heart rate, allow you to squeeze in more exercise in the same amount of time and, best of all, burn more fat. When you finish Superset 1 (the 1A and 1B sequence), rest for 45 seconds before repeating Superset 1 again.

■ Now rest for 60–75 seconds (while repeatedly telling yourself what a good job you're doing), and then do Superset 2 (exercises 2A and 2B), performing these twice, and so on, until you've completed Superset 4 twice.

■ Once you've finished this workout, do a few of your favourite stretches.

■ It's important that you attempt to perform each exercise as quickly as you can, but make sure that you carefully adhere to all the technique tips. Take it easy at first and then, when you're more familiar with the programme, really push yourself so that you break into a sweat – the higher the intensity you can work at, the better.

■ Every third to fifth workout session, shorten the break between the pairs of exercises (Supersets) by 5 seconds, so that eventually your 45-second rest is reduced to 30 seconds.

■ In Week 3, add another set to all four of the Supersets so that you're doing each Superset three times.

THE WARM-UP
1) Walk energetically on the spot, lifting your knees as high as you can and vigorously swinging your arms for 30 seconds.
2) Jog on the spot for 30 seconds.
3) Repeat steps 1 and 2 three times, with minimal rest between them.

1A BEGINNER BURPEES

'This move works your entire body, improves your flexibility and balance and even has cardio benefits,' says Coach Bronek.

a) Stand with your arms at your sides. Then crouch down, placing your hands a few centimetres in front of your feet and keeping your bodyweight distributed between your hands and feet.

b) Now rapidly extend one leg backwards so that you look as if you're waiting for the start gun in the 100m sprint (see illustration 1), followed by your other leg so that you're in a press-up position with your body in a straight line (see illustration 2).

c) Now reverse the movement, bending the leg you extended first and bringing it in towards your chest, followed by your other leg.

d) Now stand up and raise your arms straight above your head.

	EXERCISE	REPETITIONS	REST
Superset 1	**1A** Beginner burpees	10	0 secs
	1B Star jumps	30	45 secs
	60–75 seconds' rest		
Superset 2	**2A** Walking lunges with front arm raises	10 strides with each leg	0 secs
	2B Bicycle crunches	10 on each side	45 secs
	60–75 seconds' rest		
Superset 3	**3A** Iron-cross squats	20	0 secs
	3B Beginner press-ups	10	45 secs
	60–75 seconds' rest		
Superset 4	**4A** Bulgarian split squats	8–10 with each leg	0 secs
	4B Mountain climbers	10 with each leg, gradually building up to 20 with each leg	45 secs

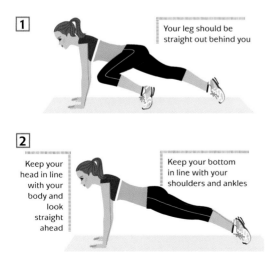

1 Your leg should be straight out behind you

2 Keep your head in line with your body and look straight ahead

Keep your bottom in line with your shoulders and ankles

1B STAR JUMPS

This is a very popular exercise with professional sports coaches and the military.

a) Stand with your feet together and your arms by your sides – this is your starting position.

b) Now jump your legs apart while simultaneously raising your arms to the sides (as illustrated) until your hands touch overhead.

c) Then jump your legs together as you lower your arms and return to your starting position.

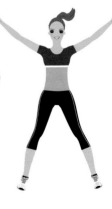

2A WALKING LUNGES WITH FRONT ARM RAISES

'Talk about multi-tasking!' says Coach Bronek. 'This exercise combines walking forwards with lunges and arm raises to make the most of every second of workout time.'

a) Stand with your arms by your sides – this is your starting position. Then take a long stride forwards with one leg while simultaneously lowering your rear knee towards the ground and raising your arms above your head (as illustrated).

b) Stop before your knee touches the ground and then, using your leg and hip muscles, push off your rear leg as you stand upright again while lowering your arms to the starting position.

c) Repeat by stepping forwards with your other leg.

2B BICYCLE CRUNCHES

'According to a study[8] of the most effective commonly performed abdominal exercises, conducted at the Biomechanics Lab at San Diego State University, this is simply the best and most effective stomach-toning exercise, which is why I've included it for you here,' says Coach Bronek. 'So forget doing hundreds of crunches – hopping on your own "body bicycle" is where it's at!'

a) Lie on your back with your hands touching either your ears or neck.

b) Now perform a 'bicycling' action with your legs by bringing one of your knees towards your chest and lifting your opposite shoulder blade off the ground so that your elbow almost touches your opposite knee (as illustrated). Your straight leg should be raised off the ground.

c) Now switch sides, bringing your other knee towards your chest and extending the knee you'd previously bent while lifting your other shoulder off the ground and trying to touch your elbow with it.

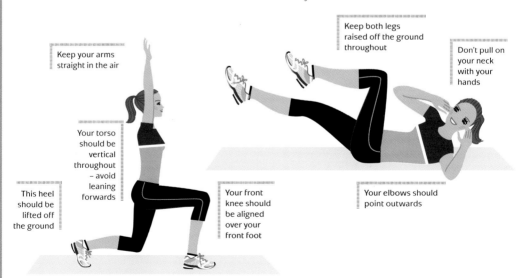

Keep your arms straight in the air

Your torso should be vertical throughout – avoid leaning forwards

This heel should be lifted off the ground

Your front knee should be aligned over your front foot

Keep both legs raised off the ground throughout

Don't pull on your neck with your hands

Your elbows should point outwards

3A IRON-CROSS SQUATS

'This squat is very similar to the squats you've been adoring doing up until now,' says Coach Bronek, 'but the addition of arm movements makes this move more challenging and enhances its overall training effect.'

a) Stand with your feet slightly wider than hip-width apart and your toes pointing slightly outwards. Hold your arms straight out to the sides.

b) Now bend at the hips and push your bottom out and backwards as you bend your knees, keeping your knees pushed apart, while lowering your bottom as low as you can (as if you're about to sit down on a chair), while simultaneously bringing your arms together in front of you (as illustrated).

c) Once you've gone as low as you can go with good technique, reverse the movement and stand upright again, while simultaneously moving your arms out to the sides.

3B BEGINNER PRESS-UPS

This version is a lot easier than conventional press-ups, so there's no excuse not to do it. Even shapelier arms, here we come!

a) Kneel on all fours and place your hands flat on the ground, slightly wider apart than your shoulders – this is your starting position. Keep your shoulders directly above your hands and your knees directly under your hips.

b) Now slowly bend your arms and lower your upper body as far as you can so that you nearly touch your chest to the ground. Aim to keep your nose forwards, well ahead of your hands (as illustrated), not directly down.

c) Now press your torso off the ground and return to your starting position.

▶ COACHING TIP FOR BEGINNER PRESS-UPS

'As you get fitter, you can make this exercise a little harder by placing your knees further back than your hips, which will shift more bodyweight onto your arms than the easier version above,' says Coach Bronek.

Keep looking at a fixed point ahead of you to stop yourself leaning forwards

Keep your arms parallel to the ground

Keep your back as upright as you can throughout the entire movement

Keep your heels down and feet flat on the ground

Keep your elbows close to your torso and avoid flaring your arms out

Keep your head in line with your torso and avoid bending your neck

4A BULGARIAN SPLIT SQUATS

By now you've probably realised that squats are Coach Bronek's most-beloved exercise. 'Make them your favourite, too, and you'll reap loads of body benefits,' he says. 'I only prescribe them because they allow you to do the most work in the least amount of time. This version not only strengthens the front of your thighs but also significantly increases your metabolic rate.'

a) Stand with your back to a bench or stool and rest the top of one foot on it. Now hop forwards a few steps with your front leg – this is your starting position.

b) Bend your front knee, going as low as you can comfortably go, ideally until your front thigh is parallel to the ground (if it isn't, hop your front leg further forwards). If you find it difficult to keep your balance, you can hold on to a lamppost, pole, broomstick or other sturdy object (as illustrated).

c) Now slowly straighten your legs until you're back in your starting position. Perform the recommended number of repetitions on one leg, and then swap legs and repeat.

Keep your torso vertical

Your knee should be at a 90° angle to the ground

4B MOUNTAIN CLIMBERS

'This is a very intense exercise,' says Coach Bronek, 'but will give you lovely, lean-looking legs and trim abs.'

a) Start this exercise as you would if you had your arms extended in a full press-up position (in other words, supporting your bodyweight with your toes and arms, with your head, torso, hips and legs in a straight line – see illustration 2 on page 109).

b) Keeping both hands on the ground, step forwards with one leg and bring that knee as close to your chest as possible (as illustrated). Then do a little hop and return that leg to your starting position while simultaneously bringing your other knee to your chest (think of it as running on the spot with your hands on the ground!).

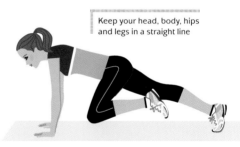

Keep your head, body, hips and legs in a straight line

> ### COACHING TIP FOR MOUNTAIN CLIMBERS
> 'Initially, do a few repetitions slowly in order to coordinate the whole move, but once you've mastered it, start speeding up,' says Coach Bronek.

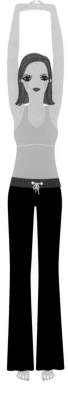

CARDIO

You continue doing moderate-intensity daily cardio (such as walking to feed those ducks or vigorous vacuuming or The Sneaky Workout) for up to 45 minutes, but now you increase the number of Power Cardio Sessions you do as part of that 45-minute activity slot to three times a week.

▶ YOUR POWER CARDIO SESSIONS

Your Power Cardio Sessions are exactly the same as in Week 6 of Six Weeks To Slim (see page 107), but now you'll be adding a minute more time to the session each week.

Warm-up 5 minutes of brisk walking or jogging.
Interval 30 seconds of high-intensity exercise (if you're walking, this means power-walking; if you're running, this means sprinting; if you're cycling, it means pedalling like mad).
Recovery 30 seconds of recovery (if you're walking, this means slower walking; if you're running, it means jogging; if you're cycling, this means pedalling sedately).
Repeat the Interval and Recovery sections 6 times.
Cool-down 5 minutes of brisk walking or jogging plus stretches.
TOTAL TIME 16 minutes of fantastic fat-burning cardio.

■ **Week 1** Do the Power Cardio Session, below left, three times a week.
■ **Week 2** Repeat the Interval and Recovery sections 7 times (a total of 17 minutes).
■ **Week 3** Repeat the Interval and Recovery sections 8 times (a total of 18 minutes).
■ **Week 4** Repeat the Interval and Recovery sections 9 times (a total of 19 minutes).
■ **Week 5** Repeat the Interval and Recovery sections 10 times (a total of 20 minutes).
■ **Week 6** Repeat the Interval and Recovery sections 10 times (a total of 20 minutes).

WHERE DO YOU GO FROM HERE?

Once you've completed both Six Weeks To Slim and Six Weeks To Super-Fit, you need to again change your programme to ensure that you keep getting fitter. At this point it would be a good idea to hire a personal trainer to write a new programme for you, or alternatively, visit Coach Bronek's website, www.coachbronek.com, where you'll find several workouts designed to follow on where these left off. Happy training!

8 WAYS TO MAKE FITNESS FUN

The lucky ones among us are born liking exercise, but for the rest of us it can be an acquired taste. No one can say they disliked exercise more than I did – I simply detested it, and associated it with embarrassment and discomfort (for more on this, see my beginner's running book, *Running Made Easy*). Forget being picked last for teams, I was so uncoordinated and slow that I was *never* picked! So how did I go from having honorary lifetime membership of the Couch Potato Society to being someone who's done 20 marathons, five triathlons and two 56-mile (89km) ultra-marathons? Well, in all honesty, I *tricked* myself into liking it by never allowing myself to get bored and continually attempting new challenges. I also made sure that all my exercise experiences were positive by seeing getting fit as a chance to gossip with my friends, to wear fancy dress (only when actually running marathons, mind!) and to boost my self-belief. I still can't quite believe that I've been exercising regularly now for 12 years – and enjoy it! Read on to find out how you, too, can change your mindset and start seeing exercise as the life-affirming activity it most certainly is.

1 I run to chat! And I'm convinced it's the main reason I'm still exercising today. Chatting makes anything seem easy, and before you know it, you're back home almost without realising you've exercised. So rope in a few friends and do anything that gets you active together. When I worked in an office, I helped to set up a twice-weekly lunchtime running club, and also proclaimed myself as my colleagues' 'personal trainer' (I had great fun bossing my boss Kate Donoughue around while teaching her the moves I'd been taught by Coach Bronek).

2 Accept that the first ten minutes of any cardio exercise are going to feel less than fabulous – I call this the 'toxic ten minutes'. However, it always gets a lot easier after that, so just grit your teeth and keep on going.

3 Ditch the 'sloth cloths' (that T-shirt you polish the car with) and invest in fab fitness gear that makes you feel good. Looking cooler than a packet of mints will make you push yourself harder as you strive to live up to your new sporty image.

4 Be a have-a-go hero! The gym isn't the only place where you can get fit – there are literally thousands of different activities you could try, from using a WiiFit to flamenco dancing to fitness

videos, trampolining to bootcamps to rock climbing to cross-country running to netball. If you don't like something, go three times, and if it's still not you, move on to the next exciting thing. I'm also told there are hundreds of apps for your mobile phone that can motivate, inform and inspire you – try them and see!

5 Treat yourself like a sporting celebrity. I keep a Fitness CV on my computer where I record details of every race I've run, along with the time I did. My loft conversion houses a display of every medal I've earned over the years, and I also have a running album showcasing my race numbers and finishing photos. All these things are a reminder that I'm now officially 'sporty'.

6 Go on adventures! Spice up your walking, running or cycling route by going somewhere you've never gone before – working out where you are on the map is all part of the fun. Or follow bus routes and see where they take you. Alternatively, aim to visit every landmark, historic building or park in your neighbourhood. Ticking off a few chores

during your workout can make it feel even more worthwhile - I often include posting letters or going to the bank in my runs.

7 Spend a day at the races. Having a race or group event to train for will give you a deadline and ensure you get out the door, no matter what it's like outside (bad weather is just an excuse for even bigger bragging rights – I've lost count of the times I've dined out on my tales of having my face exfoliated by a light hailstorm). How well you do is immaterial. I've come last (yes, really last!) in two of the five triathlons I've done, but I love the fact that I can now add 'triathlete' to the list of new words to describe myself.

8 Revel in your après-exercise. I simply adore showering after my workouts and always use an invigorating shower gel followed by a heavenly body lotion. Every day I also incorporate a different element of my beauty regime by, for example, using a face or hair mask one day and filing my nails the next. By the end of the week I've taken care of every single part of my body and feel like a million dollars, ready for the weekend.

HYPNOTISE YOURSELF SLIM: TRACK 3

Now it's time to start using hypnosis as your Secret Slimming Tool to increase your fitness motivation and help you to appreciate the exhilarating, mood-boosting benefits of exercise. Find a quiet place where you won't be disturbed, sit back, relax and listen to Track 3 (Exercise Yourself Slim) on your hypnosis CD (turn back to page 82 for more detailed instructions on how to do this). At the end of this ten-minute hypnosis session you'll awaken feeling fully energised and raring to experience how great it feels to be getting fitter. Alternate this track with Track 2, aiming to listen to each of them once a day (preferably first thing in the morning and last thing at night) as you continue on your way to Destination Dream Weight.

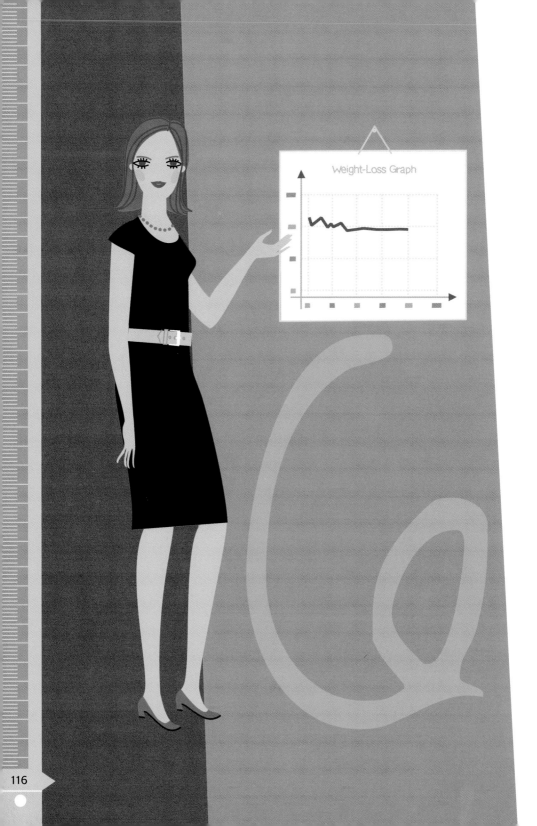

Weight-Loss Graph

Chapter 6

Get yourself OVER A PLATEAU

You've been doing brilliantly and then, out of the blue, the pounds stubbornly refuse to budge. Don't despair! Or beat yourself up. Plateaus are a very normal part of weight management, so don't let them throw you off course. With these tried-and-tested techniques and success-guaranteed strategies, you'll be able to work out what's gone wrong and develop your own set of problem-solving skills

THE PLATEAU UNCOVERED

If your weight has stayed the same for at least three to four weeks, this means your body is in energy balance, according to Lyndel. In other words, the calories you're consuming are in balance with how many you're burning. It's very normal to get 'change fatigue' and slip back into old habits or eat that bit more than you realise. 'Keep filling in your *Adore Yourself Slim* Travel Journal, especially the food diary sections, and look back to see how it compares with what you were eating when you were losing weight, says Lyndel. 'You may notice extra snacks sneaking in, larger portion sizes, or that you've been eating out more. Check, too, whether your level of activity has slipped a bit. Aim to get back to past helpful habits. And do a reality check to see if there's something going on in your life at the moment that's making it more difficult for you to follow your plan. It may also be a sign that it's time to investigate if any (often unconscious) thoughts and feelings are stopping you from making the changes you want.'

Usually this will be enough to get you moving again. 'However,' says Lyndel, 'if you've addressed all these things and have already lost at least 2st (12.7kg), but your weight hasn't budged for a month or so, then you may need to adjust your diet or exercise levels a bit. Now that you're lighter, there's less of you burning energy (calories) day to day. Ideally, start with an increase in exercise. If you need more of a boost, then reduce your Snacks/Extras servings from daily to twice a week (or, if you're following a different eating plan to ours, cut back about 100 calories a day). Meanwhile, remember that sometimes we need to have a rest from active weight loss for a while, and just get used to maintaining it, before feeling ready to move on.'

THE IMPORTANCE OF HAPPY TALK

Our automatic thoughts (or self-talk) have a real influence on how we feel and act. Take negative thoughts about body image as an example. If you're deeply dissatisfied with your body, negative thoughts can take over. This dissatisfaction can reach beyond just wanting to lose some weight into a deeper dislike of yourself, triggering the need for something comforting. This often leads to overeating – and further

66 Use the STOP technique to evict the Wicked Witch who fills your mind with negative self-talk 99

negative self-talk ('I've blown it, I fail at everything, I'm not worth the effort, I may as well give up…'). And so the cycle of negative emotions leading to negative behaviours leading to negative emotions continues. Automatic thoughts usually develop over the course of a lifetime, so can be stubborn. One way to deal with persistent negative self-talk is to use the STOP technique (see Evict the Wicked Witch on page 32).

ANALYSING THE PROS AND CONS OF WEIGHT LOSS

Being slimmer has plenty of plus sides, but what many women don't realise is that there can also be downsides: slimming can interfere with your social life, for example, because you can't go out for boozy girls' nights quite so often; or it can take more time to plan and cook meals. Even if you think you're desperate to lose weight, you may not be consciously aware of the things that may be blocking your progress. Hidden reasons for maintaining negative or unhelpful behaviours are called 'secondary gains' and they arise because your unconscious mind is trying to protect you from things that it perceives to be potentially harmful. The way to uncover these secondary gains is to ask yourself what you're gaining by not losing weight, as once you've identified your motivation to stay overweight, you can address these underlying issues and move forward again. Use the chart below to help you do this. If you decide that the Pros outweigh the Cons, you're ready to get cracking with your plateau-busting plan (see What Lisa Did, overleaf). Remember to use the information you've gathered in your Cons list to plan how you're going to overcome these potential obstacles to success. If you find that the Cons outweigh the Pros, this may not be the best time to actively lose weight, so aim to maintain the changes you've already made, take it easy and try this exercise again in a month or so.

HOW I CURRENTLY FEEL ABOUT LOSING WEIGHT

PROS (I'll feel more energetic/ sexier; I'll be able to fit into my clothes; I'll feel more confident and in control, etc)

CONS (I'll have to limit eating out; I'll have to plan more; I may attract unwanted sexual attention; I won't get comfort from junk food, etc)

When I'd been following my new healthy lifestyle for about two months, I hit a plateau. All of a sudden my once-friendly scales stopped smiling at me and got stuck at 11st 11lb (75kg) and my motivation (and faith in the eating plan) started to wane. After a couple of weeks of yo-yoing around this weight, I decided to hold a Personal Slimming Summit and find out what was going on. So I sat down and took a detailed look at what I was doing and, surprise, surprise, found that my plateau was far from inexplicable. When I was honest with myself, I realised that I'd started to backslide in many small but important ways. I was no longer religiously doing my self-hypnosis on the train every morning (nor was I doing The Sneaky Workout or regularly rewarding myself), I'd got out of the routine of going food shopping on a Monday (and as a result I was cooking food I didn't really like from whatever I could find in the kitchen, which meant I also ate high-calorie foods to compensate) and I was frequently omitting to weigh and measure myself. With these findings to hand, I set about rediscovering my enthusiasm for the programme by:

■ reading every compliment I'd received up to that point (see page 146) and looking back on my progress as evidenced by my dipping Weight-Loss Graph (see page 52).
■ revisiting what I loved about myself and what others loved about me (see page 9), and what I adored about my body (see The *Adore Yourself Slim* Body Map on page 34).
■ recalling my Body Scan (see page 30) to remind me how I used to feel when I was 2st 1lb (13.3kg) heavier – the weight of my fully-packed travelling backpack – and how breathless I used to get walking up a flight of stairs; how uncomfortable many of my clothes felt.
■ reminding myself that I had a Goal Group (see page 36) of friends, family and experts who were all willing me to succeed.
■ looking back to my reasons to be slim (see page 46) and finding new short-, medium- and long-term benefits to getting to my goal

HYPNOTISE YOURSELF OVER A PLATEAU: TRACK 4

When I'm working with my hypnotherapy patients, I often ask them to imagine what their life would be like six months from now if they made the changes they say they want to make, and also what things would be like if they decided not to change. If you want to use hypnosis as a Secret Slimming Tool to help you analyse whether this is the best time to continue losing weight or whether you need to wait a while before recommitting to adoring yourself slim, listen to Track 4 on your hypnosis CD now (and then fill in the chart opposite). The track is also designed to reinforce the plateau-busting strategies mentioned in this chapter, and to reinspire and remotivate you. Listen to it at least once a day in addition to either Track 2 or 3 until you've got over the plateau, then revert to listening to Tracks 2 and 3 daily until you reach Destination Dream Weight, when it'll be time to switch to Track 5.

IF I DON'T MAKE LIFESTYLE CHANGES NOW, HOW WILL I FEEL IN SIX MONTHS' TIME?

POSITIVES
(I won't have had to worry about failing; I'll still be able to socialise and eat out a lot; I'll feel safe, etc)

_____
_____
_____
_____
_____
_____
_____
_____
_____
_____
_____
_____

NEGATIVES
(I'll probably have gained even more weight; I'll feel sluggish; I'll feel I've let myself down, etc)

_____
_____
_____
_____
_____
_____
_____
_____
_____
_____
_____
_____

weight, plus reviewing my Ten Slimming Commandments (see page 74) and my Want-To-Do List (see page 55), and adding a few more exciting things I wanted to do before I died (wear jeans again, go rock climbing, try Rollerblading, run the 56-mile/ 89km Comrades ultra-marathon).

■ vowing to resume grocery shopping on a Monday and to challenge myself to find new, flavour-packed recipes (see page 84) to keep my meals interesting.

■ recommitting to all my new healthy habits (see the Adoption Certificate on page 83): sitting on a Swiss ball at work, doing The Sneaky Workout (see page 99) and investigating adventurous new fitness

activities, such as triathlons (see page 114), practising self-hypnosis, getting more sleep, cutting back on alcohol and regularly weighing and measuring myself.

■ following the eating plan more closely and watching my portion sizes.

■ combating comfort eating by asking myself: 'What do I _really_ need right now?'

■ religiously filling in my _Adore Yourself Slim_ Travel Journal (see page 148), especially the sections on what I felt grateful for, the slip-ups I could learn from and the rewards I promised myself.

And, I'm happy to report, it worked, and my Weight-Loss Graph resumed its downward trend once more.

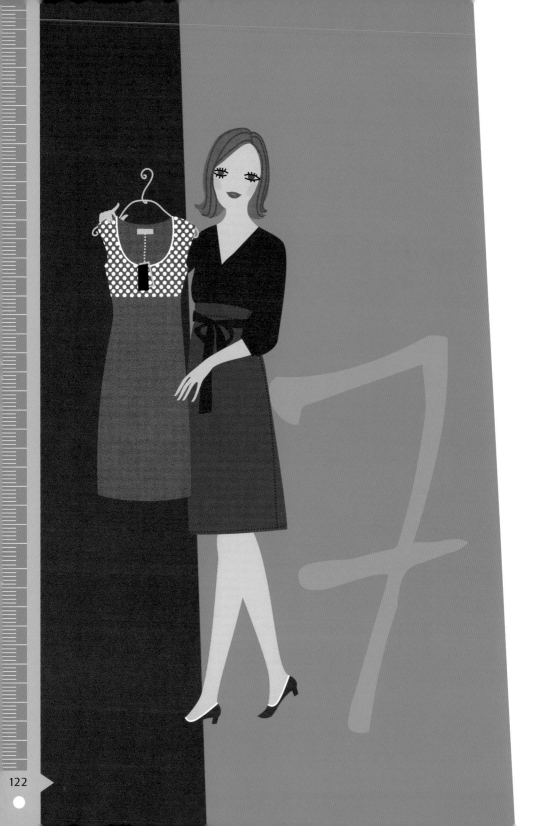

Chapter 7

DRESS yourself SLIM

And now it's time for the really, really fun bit! Today's the day when you're going to start revamping your look, from the outside in. One of the biggest mistakes many of my weight-loss patients make is to put off buying new clothes and to see shopping as a dreaded chore rather than an exercise in self-celebration (as their slimmer sisters do). They also often fail to take full advantage of the face-flattering effects of make-up. But I believe that any woman, whether she's a size 8 or 28, can be full-on fabulous, depending on the effort she's prepared to put into looking good...

DRESS TO IMPRESS

Every woman has a figure that, with the help of some clever styling and shapewear, can be turned from dumpy and dowdy into drop-dead gorgeous, which is why we're now going to turn our attention to your wardrobe. 'But,' I hear you cry, 'I'm going to be losing weight and so anything I buy now won't fit me in a few weeks' time.' Yes, that's true, but life's too short to spend even a few weeks feeling less than 100% fantastic about your appearance, so you really do need to commit to buying a few clothes at every stage of your weight-loss journey. While you're slimming it's sensible to buy less-expensive outfits, but whatever you do, don't put off buying clothes altogether – nothing's going to inspire you to stick with this programme more than looking your best right here, right now, every single day. It's also vital to get rid of any clothes that no longer fit you the minute they become too baggy. Holding on to oversized clothes tells your unconscious mind that you need an insurance plan just in case this programme doesn't work for you, which sets you up for failure. Don't delay – take those ill-fitting clothes to that charity shop today.

GOING FROM GLUM TO GLAM

During my own weight-loss journey, I realised that years of taking a 'I-can't-be-bothered' attitude to fashion because I was overweight meant I knew next to nothing about it, and so I turned to an ex-colleague, Jayne Ellis of Reinvent My Style.com, for advice. Jayne works for ELLE magazine as an advertising manager, but runs a styling business in her spare time, and her passion for fashion is infectious. Jayne reminded me that all of us have attractive features that are worth celebrating, and that instead of obsessing about the parts of our body we don't like, we should focus on making the most of those we do. So here's how to go about doing that…

STEP 1: DECIDE ON YOUR LOOK

To do this, you need to choose what image you want to portray at work and when socialising or at home (so you'll need to choose more than one).

- ■ Professional/sophisticated ❑
- ■ Casual/sporty/sexy ❑
- ■ Cool/trendy/quirky ❑

Next, find examples of women who already have the look you're aiming for and ask yourself *how* they've achieved it. So, for example, if you want to look 'professional', find someone who embodies that look (a work colleague?; a news reader?), then keep your eyes peeled on the bus/train/high street for ideas and scan magazines and newspapers to analyse the key elements that make the look work (eg skirt length, colours, shoe style), and write down your observations here.

_____

_____

_____

STEP 2: CUPBOARD CLEANSE

In exactly the same way that you eliminated 'toxic' foodstuffs from your kitchen, you now need to perform a clothing clear-out. The easiest way to ease your wardrobe worries is to sort your clothes into two piles:

a) Clothes you never wear Go through each item and tick the reasons why you don't wear it below. This will give you an understanding of what hasn't worked for you in the past and will prove invaluable when you go shopping.

■ It doesn't fit properly on my (jot down where the item doesn't fit)

_____

_____

■ It's unflattering because

_____

■ It's dated ❏
■ The colour (list which ones) doesn't suit me

_____

_____

■ The length (list which ones) doesn't suit me

_____

_____

■ It needs to be... hand-washed ❏
ironed ❏
dry-cleaned ❏
and I can never be bothered to do that.
■ I don't have anything to wear with it ❏

The latter is the only item that may need a rethink before you ditch it – try to work out what will make that item work (a better bra, cardie, jacket, belt?), write it down above and then take this book with you when you go clothes shopping and see whether you can find whatever's missing to rehabilitate the item back into your wardrobe.

ITEM THAT ISN'T WORKING	WHAT I NEED TO BUY TO MAKE IT WORK

Then put all these items into charity bags and either give them away immediately or, if you're convinced you'll grieve for your unloved things, store them in the loft or shed for a year. If you haven't missed anything you've thrown out during that time, donate the (unopened) bags to charity.

b) Clothes you wear all the time Sort everything by category so that all your tops, trousers, jackets and so on are hanging together in your wardrobe. While you're doing this, think about why you love every item. Really try to understand why you wear what you wear all the time. How does it make you feel? Is it easy to wear? Maybe it's just safe and you now realise that that's no longer enough for you (in which case, consign it to your charity-bag pile)? Then ask yourself if this really is how you want to continue dressing for the rest of your life. If the answer is 'Yes, I love this stuff – it's soooo me! I look fabulous!', then you really don't need to read this section of the book. If not, read on!

Now use the chart overleaf to carry out a stock-take so that when you hit the shops you'll know exactly what you need to buy to fill in any gaps in your wardrobe.

THE SAVVY SHOPPER'S CLOTHES SHOPPING LIST

ITEM	HOW MANY YOU'VE GOT	HOW MANY YOU NEED TO BUY/ COLOUR	STYLING DETAILS YOU NEED TO LOOK OUT FOR (SEE STEP 5, OVERLEAF)
Trousers			
Jeans			
Suits			
Shirts			
Blouses/T-shirts			
Skirts			
Coats			
Casual dresses			
Smart dresses			
Jumpers/cardigans/ polo-necks			
Coats			
Jackets/blazers			
Shoes			
Flats			
Heels			
Boots			
Swimwear			
Sportswear			
Accessories/jewellery			
Underwear			
Bras			
Knickers			
Support underwear			
Tights/leggings			

STEP 3: WORK OUT YOUR COLOUR PALETTE

Next, you need to work out which colours suit you. Remember, white compliments your face as it illuminates your skin. Black does the reverse, so as you get older, opt for navy instead because it's slightly softer. Once you've seen what white can do for your skin, hold up other colours to your face and see if they have a positive or negative effect on your skin tone. If in doubt, ask a friend round and colour match together.

The colours that suit me are

_____

_____

_____

_____

_____

_____

_____

The colours that
don't do anything
for me are

_____

_____

_____

_____

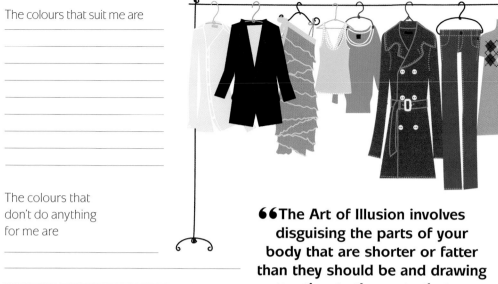

❝The Art of Illusion involves disguising the parts of your body that are shorter or fatter than they should be and drawing attention to the parts that are smaller and slimmer❞

STEP 4: ANALYSE YOUR BODY

Only a tiny number of women actually have a perfectly proportioned body that's the exact shape and size of the clothes in shops, hence the long queues you tend to find in changing rooms and at the refund desk. The reason that some women look good and others don't is because some women understand the 'Art of Illusion', which involves, yes, you guessed it, creating the *illusion* that they have a perfectly proportioned body. This is done very simply by disguising the parts of your body that are shorter, fatter or wider than they (conventionally) should be, and by drawing attention to the parts that are smaller, slimmer or narrower (and that you're secretly quite pleased with). I'd like you now to take a long, hard look at yourself naked in a full-length mirror and fill in what you consider to be your lovely body bits (look back to your Body Map on page 34 for ideas) and your not-so-lovely body bits…

I LOVE MY GORGEOUS…

Slender neck	❏	Small waist	❏
Big boobs	❏	Flat tummy	❏
Small boobs	❏	Narrow hips	❏
Shoulders	❏	Pert bottom	❏
Back	❏	Long legs	❏
Toned arms	❏	Shapely ankles	❏
Slender wrists	❏	Feet	❏
Hands	❏		

ER… I'M NOT REALLY ON SPEAKING TERMS WITH MY…

Flat chest	❏	Jelly belly	❏
Big boobs	❏	Wide hips	❏
Wobbly upper arms	❏	Big bottom	❏
Wide waist	❏	Chunky thighs	❏

STEP 5: START PERFECTING THE ART OF ILLUSION

Now it's time to make the most of your assets and balance out or disguise your less-than-perfect bits by choosing the styles that suit your body shape. With these simple style rules, anyone can look truly amazing at any weight...

▶ HOW TO BALANCE OUT A FLAT CHEST

Polo-necks Tight ones will make your bust look bigger – but avoid them if you have a short neck. Skinny polo-necks are especially good for pear-shaped women who have a small waist, as they make your bust look bigger and cling to your slender waist.

A good bra There are some amazing padded bras available, but if you really want to add a bit of extra volume, opt for a gel-filled one. Also consider wearing 'chicken fillets' inside your bra.

Other styles that suit you Frilled or ruffled shirts; double-breasted jackets; horizontal stripes; brightly coloured and bold patterned tops.

▶ HOW TO DISGUISE WOBBLY UPPER ARMS

Long sleeves These should be your first choice. Opt for capped sleeves or elbow-length shirts as a summer option. Remember that fake tan will make your upper arms look slimmer.

Other styles that suit you Bolero jackets; cardies; shrugs.

Avoid at all costs Spaghetti straps; strapless tops; sleeveless T-shirts; halterneck tops or dresses.

▶ HOW TO BALANCE OUT BIG BOOBS

Fitted shirts These should always fit perfectly around your bust area, even if they gape at your waist. If you find that shirts don't fit your waist, either get them altered or belt them, but be careful – a waist that's overly nipped-in can make big boobs look bigger.

Other styles that suit you V-necks; chokers (only opt for these if you have a longish neck, as they make short necks look shorter); shirts with narrow lapels; single-breasted jackets and coats.

Avoid at all costs Big patterns and bold colours on your top half; polo-necks.

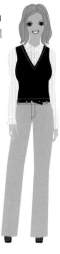

▶ HOW TO BALANCE OUT A WIDE WAIST

Dropped waists These work especially well if you have a wider waist, as they draw the eye to your narrow hips while concealing the fact that you don't have much of a waistline.

Other styles that suit you Low-slung belts; straight-legged trousers; dresses and tops that feature ruching around the middle.

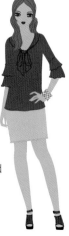

▶ HOW TO DISGUISE A JELLY BELLY

Empire line This style flares from just below your bust, thus highlighting the narrowest part of your body and hiding a jelly belly or wide waist.

Dropped waists These create a belt effect and draw attention to your hips, but they only work if your hips are (proportionally) narrow.

Other styles that suit you Loose-fitted shift dresses; dresses and tops with ruching or draping around the middle (with the latter, the observer can't work out if it's your tummy or the fabric that's creating a slight curve!); long jackets over above-the-knee dresses.

Avoid at all costs Tight belts; very fitted jackets, shirts and dresses.

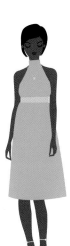

▶ HOW TO DISGUISE A BIG BOTTOM

Cleverly placed back pockets These will instantly lift your derrière, making it look more pert.

A-line dresses and skirts These not only disguise a big bottom but draw attention to your slim waist or legs.

Anything that builds up your top half Bulkier clothes on your upper body will make your bottom appear smaller.

Other styles that suit you Dark trousers and skirts.

Avoid at all costs High-waisted trousers; light colours or large prints on your bottom half as this will draw attention to it.

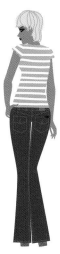

▶ HOW TO BALANCE OUT WIDE HIPS

Big shoulders Anything that widens your shoulders (such as epaulettes, shoulder pads or puffed sleeves) will, by contrast, make your hips look narrower.

Tailored jackets with a wide shoulder and nipped-in waist These can balance out wider hips, as they tend to draw the eye upwards to the waistline while the built-up shoulder line balances out your hips.

Other styles that suit you Bootleg and tailored trousers; A-line skirts and dresses.

Avoid at all costs Bulk on your widest part (gathers and pleats, and also bulky, thick materials, such as wool and tweed); dropped waists (they draw attention to your hips); anything too tight around your hips.

▶ HOW TO BALANCE OUT CHUNKY THIGHS

A-line skirts They disguise the shape or size of your thighs and show off pretty ankles.

Bootcut jeans and trousers These help to balance larger thighs by kicking out slightly at the knee.

Wide-legged trousers Wear with a fitted top/jacket, as volume on the bottom half needs to be balanced by tailoring on the top, and vice versa. Always wear with a heel or wedge.

Other styles that suit you Dark-coloured trousers and denim; double-breasted jackets.

Avoid at all costs Skinny jeans; light-coloured trousers.

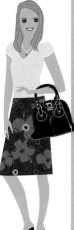

YOUR WARDROBE ESSENTIALS

▶ JEANS

Jeans are the number-one, can't-live-without item of clothing as they work for so many different events, from smart-casual (team with a white shirt and blazer) to an evening out with the girls (add heels and a sparkly top) to that oh-so stressful first/second/third date (worn with a low heel boot and a cute Tee/vest). They can also make you look younger and/or fashionable and send out the message: 'I haven't tried too hard to look this good!'. Always try to get a snug fit because a well-fitting pair of jeans can be like a plunge bra for the bottom – they'll lift your buttocks and push them together, instantly creating a pert derrière. Believe it or not, there is a pair out there for everyone, but you need to be prepared to devote an entire shopping trip (or even three, according to Jayne!) solely to searching out the perfect jeans.

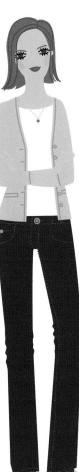

Jeans are possibly the least-standardised item of clothing when it comes to size as they vary according to the brand, cut and how stretchy they are. It's easier if you decide what you're looking for before you start shopping (black wide-legged or skinny stonewash, for example) as this will help to refine your search, but it can also be fun experimenting with different styles. The most flattering jeans are dark denim bootcut. And don't be afraid to try stretch denim (ideally, it should say 2% elastane or Lycra/Spandex on the label), which makes everyone look slimmer but is especially good for pear shapes because it fits a small waist while also stretching to accommodate wider hips and a bigger bottom.

▶ WHITE SHIRT

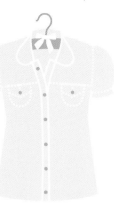

A perfectly fitted white shirt is a wardrobe winner. The colour instantly lifts most skin tones and it works just as well for weekendwear (worn with jeans it can look smart-casual) as it does for officewear (wear it with a smart pair of trousers and a tailored jacket). And best of all, there's one to suit every bodyshape: go for high collared if you have a long neck, ruffles if you have small boobs, puff sleeves if you have narrow shoulders or tailored if you have a wide waist.

▶ TAILORED JACKET

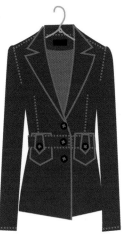

This works wonders when you want to feel instantly smart. Buy one that compliments your body shape (see the previous page). Only wear long (below the bottom) jackets if you've got long legs – they'll create the illusion of a longer torso.

▶ NUDE SHOES

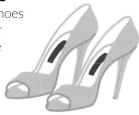

Nude-coloured shoes blend in with your skin, and because you can't tell where your legs end and your feet begin, they instantly make your legs look longer. In addition, nude is a neutral colour and therefore can be worn with pretty much any colour or outfit.

▶ BLACK TROUSERS

Simply everyone needs a pair of black trousers! Not only do they go with most things but they're appropriate for most occasions and make your legs look longer, your hips and bottom smaller and your thighs slimmer. As there are so many styles out there, here's a guide to choosing the perfect pair…

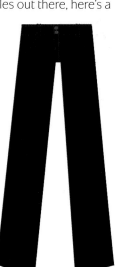

■ **Bootcut and wide legged** Best for pear shapes as the gentle flare balances out wider hips (but ideally wear with heels!)

■ **Straight leg** Best if you've got a boyish figure because if you have a curvy figure they can make your hips look wider.

■ **Tapered or skinny** Only opt for these if you don't mind adding width to your hips! As these trousers go in at the ankle, they tend to create the illusion that your hips are wider than they really are.

▶ UNDERWEAR
Bras

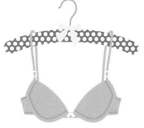

■ Always, always, always get measured professionally. There's no point in having great boobs in the wrong place (i.e. around your waist). Many high-street and department stores offer a free bra-measuring service with no pressure to buy.

■ Every woman needs a nude-coloured, seamless bra for wearing under T-shirts, white shirts, skinny polo-necks and clingy jumpers. Don't wear lacy and patterned bras under transparent or white shirts – they look dated.

■ Like good sisters, your boobs should be as close as possible, so aim for cleavage when choosing a bra.

Knickers

I used to think of supportive underwear in terms of girdles, corsets and big pants – in other words, the stuff grannies wore – and so steered clear of it. How wrong I was. When I finally decided to give shapewear a go, I was blown away by the results. That little tummy bump that no number of crunches could eliminate? Gone in an instant! Having recently tried on the most fabulous silhouette-sculpting bandage dress with – and without – a tummy-and-thigh shaper, I can honestly say that it's the best possible investment any woman could make. And nowadays, shapewear is designed to be sexy, too. It's a lot more expensive than the conventional kind, but you can wear normal knickers underneath, so you won't need to wash it every time you wear it.

STEP 6: LET'S GO SHOPPING!

At last you're ready to shop till you… look drop-dead gorgeous! Before you hit the high street armed with The Savvy Shopper's Clothes Shopping List (see page 126), read the following tips to make sure you return home with items you'll treasure for ever rather than ones you'll stash unworn at the bottom of your wardrobe.

1 **Always shop solo.** You really need to concentrate when shopping and a friend will only distract you or force you into making hasty purchases because she or he's getting bored.

2 **Always make sure you're well-watered and fed before you go out** – and only shop when you're in a good mood, as feeling less than 100% positive will affect the way you feel about every outfit.

3 **Never shop with unwashed hair or without wearing at least a little make-up** – you need to look as good as you possibly can when faced with unforgiving changing-room lighting. Take along a comb or hairbrush

and some lipstick and give yourself little touch-ups between each outfit change. Applying a body moisturiser with fake tan for a few days before you hit the shops will also boost your body confidence.

4 **Always shop in comfortable shoes or trainers,** as clocking up a lot of mall miles can play havoc with your feet and make you want to head for home long before you've accomplished your shopping objectives. However, never forget to bring along the underwear, accessories and shoes you envisage wearing with what you're hunting for (if you've forgotten them at home, find something similar in the store you're in and try them on along with potential purchases).

5 **Never be too shy to consult the shop assistants** – they're the experts and know their stock inside out. Use The Savvy Shopper's Clothes Shopping List and avoid the time-wasting chore of wading through the rails by asking for help in finding what you need. Save even more time by asking the assistants to fetch you different sizes, or to suggest alternatives when trying things on.

LISA'S LOOK-GOOD RULES

1 Be posture perfect You only have to look at magazines to see how key posture is for celebs when they want to present a confident, stylish image. Good posture will make you look slimmer and more confident and, best of all, it's free (which means more money to shop!). Take a few moments now to think about what your current posture says about you – remember it's the first thing we notice about each other, especially when meeting for the first time, and it's even more important than how you dress! Good posture is pretty straightforward: keep your shoulders back, your head high and your tummy and bottom in. If that's too much to remember, focus on pulling in the part of your stomach under your belly button. When you first try to change your posture it may feel awkward, especially if you're used to hunching your shoulders, slouching or looking down. But please, please persist and, with practice, good posture will come more naturally and will even make you healthier as it'll help to prevent back problems.

2 Get a shoe that fits Never, never, never, regardless of how beautiful or expensive or perfectly coordinated they are, struggle around in shoes you can't walk in – it doesn't look good… and it hurts. When buying new shoes, keep the price label on the sole and wear them at home for at least two hours to see how they fit. If they hurt you or come off your feet as you walk around, take them back immediately and get a refund. Avoid wearing brand new shoes to your first date/job interview/night out with the girls, as without testing them at home first you can't possibly know if they'll be comfortable. Another tip: to avoid confidence-sapping sweaty feet, always opt for leather uppers.

3 Be well-heeled There's a reason that you so rarely see flats on the catwalk – heels make your legs look longer and your body look slimmer, and they make you feel both more professional and attractive. My biggest discovery in my fashion journey was that I could wear heels, as for decades I'd shunned them in favour of trainers or practical flats. Interestingly, it was Sarah Maxwell (the personal trainer who devised this book's Sneaky Workout) who insisted I try on her wedged heels while I was interviewing her for an article about body confidence. I'd always struggled to walk in heels, but wedged heels offer a lot more stability than stilettos – and make you feel amazing.

4 Never settle for second best Avoid buying anything just because it's cheap or you're in the mood to spend money. If something's less than perfect, ask yourself if taking it to a tailor is going to fix it (and also if you're really prepared to go to that hassle and expense). If the answer's 'No', put it back straight away. There will always be other outfits with your name on them – and you're worth the effort of seeking them out. Buy something you're less than happy with and it'll always be Plan B when you're choosing an outfit, and so you'll probably never or seldom wear it. Which will mean that on a cost-per-wear basis it'll become the most expensive item in your wardrobe – rather than that blink-and-you'll-miss-it bargain you thought you just had to snatch up.

HOW TO MAKE THE MOST OF YOURSELF

Now that you've revamped your wardrobe, it's time to turn your attention to your beauty routine. Helena Rubinstein, the founder of a global cosmetics company, once famously said, 'There are no ugly women, only lazy ones', and I believe she was right. Looking good does take time, but the results will more than repay your efforts. And once again, don't wait until you're well on the road to slimming success – wave that magic mascara wand over your life right from the word go and the increased confidence you'll feel will give you the motivation boost you need to keep going when the going gets tough.

LISA'S FAST-TRACK WAYS TO GLOW

Cleanse Firmly massage Liz Earle Cleanse & Polish Hot Cloth Cleanser, a eucalyptus and rosemary-scented cream, into (rather than onto) your skin for the ultimate deep-cleansing, circulation-boosting beauty ritual. Wipe it off with a muslin cloth rinsed in warm water and your skin will feel convent-girl clean.

Exfoliate Use an exfoliator on your body and face whenever your skin needs extra pampering attention.

Moisturise I love double-duty products, so opt for moisturisers that contain self-tan (and have a high SPF) whenever I want to have skin that looks as if it's lit from within.

Indulge Regular little treats such as facials, face masks, pedicures and manicures (or even doing your own nails) will not only make you look groomed and feel confident but will send a message to your unconscious mind that you're worth investing in. And this, in turn, will strengthen your resolve to stay on course with your weight loss.

THE TOP 4 MAKE-UP BAG MUST-HAVES

1 **Mascara** I'm a huge fan of Maybelline Pulse Perfection Vibrating Mascara, whose vibrating wand gives delightfully defined lashes with no clumping whatsoever (plus a lovely smile from being tickled!). In all my years of trialling mascaras for free while working in women's magazines, I've never come across a better one.

2 **Eyeshadow** I swear by Urban Decay, which features fab, vibrant colours in its palettes along with sparkly shadows that look like crushed glitter (a lot more grown-up than ordinary glitter shadows, but just as much fun). Match your shadow to your eyes and complexion, not your outfit, using this handy guide (though bear in mind that these aren't set in stone – just combinations that look particularly stunning).

Green and hazel eyes Dark green; deep purple; plum; soft violet; golden and greyish brown; soft peach; gold.

Blue eyes Warm brown; greyish-brown; charcoal; purple; pink; soft peach; silver; gold.

Grey eyes Purple; charcoal; cool brown.

Brown eyes Lucky you! You get to choose any gorgeous colour you want!

3 **Lipstick** I prefer lipsticks that act as lipstains because they last longer. My favourite is Maybelline, but MAC and Bobbi Brown are good, too, though pricier. Colouring in your lips with lip liner before applying lipstick or lipgloss is another top tip.

4 **Cream blusher** My beauty editor friend Alex raves about blusher – she says it's the one thing that makes you look perkier, healthier and prettier. Super-affordable Maybelline Dream Mousse Blush is her top tip.

YOUR SECRET BODY-CONFIDENCE TOOLKIT

■ When massaged in with a long-handled bath brush, zesty-and-oh-so-zingy grapefruit body scrub leaves your skin feeling smooth and kitten-soft.

■ A tanned body looks healthier and slimmer, so apply a body moisturiser that contains self-tan.

■ Dry, cracked heels are probably the biggest body beauty crime you can commit, so for kissable feet (literally overnight!), use a foot file and then apply some heel cream before popping on some socks and heading off to bed.

■ While I was losing weight I chose Elizabeth Arden's Sunflowers as my slimming scent, and every time I smelled its sunny, holiday-happy scent it reminded me of how good I was going to look on the beach if I kept going.

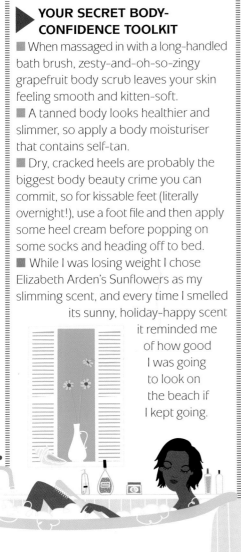

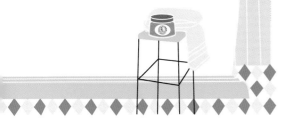

HOW TO HAVE HEAVENLY HAIR

According to hairdressers I've spoken to over the years, miscommunication is the biggest obstacle to creating the ideal hairstyle that suits both your appearance and lifestyle. To avoid this, take along at least five pictures of the styles you think might suit you (tear them out of magazines, print them off the internet or dig out old photos of yourself when you had your most flattering cut). It's also helpful if you show your stylist pictures of fringes, lengths or styles that you definitely want to avoid. And make sure you've answered the questions below before you go – and then convey this vital information to your stylist.

■ **Are you prepared to blow-dry/curl/straighten your hair every day or are you looking for a wash-and-go cut?**

_____

■ **How long are you prepared to spend on styling your hair every day?**

_____

■ **How frequently are you prepared to get your hair cut or coloured?**

_____

■ **Do you want to colour or highlight your hair or keep it natural?**

_____

■ **How does your hair react to products? Does it go limp and lanky if you use mousse, for example?**

_____

Finally, ask your stylist to explain how he or she is drying or styling your hair (and take notes if you have to). Often, more than 50% of the effect of a new cut is down to the way it's been styled, not just the cut itself.

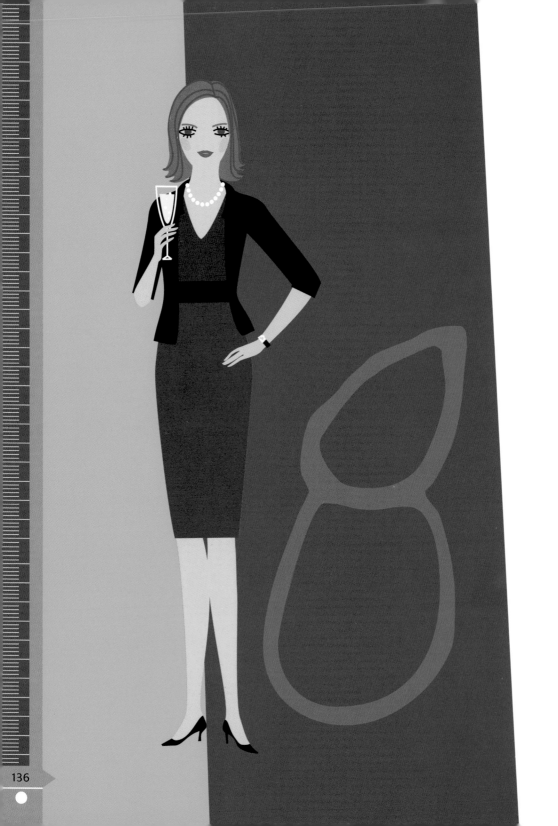

Chapter 8

Celebrate your SLIM SELF

Now's the moment you've been waiting for – it's time to pour yourself a glass of icy-cold bubbly to celebrate how truly fabulous it feels to reach Destination Dream Weight. Congratulations! You truly are amazing! But while you're savouring the warm glow of success, it's also important to use this wonderful sense of achievement to motivate yourself to keep going, because weight management is a lifelong journey, not just a short day trip. So read on to discover how the decidedly doable Stay Slim Plan allows you to eat more but stay slim, for life…

STAY SLIM FOR GOOD

You finally got there! All your hard work's been worth it and you're now the healthy weight you dreamt of being. However, before you close the book that's been your constant companion throughout this journey, don't neglect to read this chapter on how to make sure you don't regain the weight you've lost. Because if you return to your old unhelpful habits, you'll be back to square one – and we promised each other we wouldn't go there! So it's vital to remember that you need to keep using the skills and strategies you honed while slimming. Keeping the weight off can be tricky, as by now the novelty of this programme will have worn off, but the good news is that it's far easier to psyche yourself up to lose a couple of pounds (especially now that you have the skill set to do so) than it is to get in the right mindset to lose a significant amount of weight.

So what's the best way to ensure you keep adoring your slimmer self? Well, according to Lyndel, there are a host of studies[1] pointing to the things successful slimmers continue doing to maintain their weight. To give you some ideas, I've listed what the research shows, right. Of course, different things work for different people, so it's important that you find your own Secret Stay-Slim Weapons and continue to use them consistently in the weeks, months and years ahead.

THE SECRET STAY-SLIM WEAPONS

According to numerous studies, those who lose weight, and keep it off…

■ accept that remaining slim takes ongoing commitment, stay realistic and keep believing that the changes they have chosen to make are worth it.

■ eat a healthy, lower-fat diet with more fruit and vegetables.

■ incorporate daily activity into their lifestyle.

■ self-monitor – they check their weight regularly and keep (mental or written) tabs on what they eat and how active they are.

■ take action to lose weight if they regain 5lb (2.3kg).

■ eat breakfast – and regular meals, including on the weekends.

■ cook at home more and limit their consumption of fast food.

■ sit down and pay attention to what they eat, including their portion sizes.

■ practise flexible restraint (see pages 61-62) and don't feel like a failure if they do overeat or go off course.

■ watch less TV!

■ develop problem-solving skills, including finding better ways to cope with stress.

■ keep up ongoing support and accountability (that's your Goal Group).

■ find it becomes easier after two years – hurrah!

MAKE FRIENDS WITH YOUR SCALES

People who successfully remain slim after losing weight tend to continue weighing themselves at least once a week, according to Lyndel. Having gone for years without owning a set of scales, I know exactly how vital this type of self-monitoring is. If you weigh yourself regularly (or instead frequently try on a tight-fitting item of clothing), then you'll quickly notice if you've gained any weight and can take prompt action to lose it again. Checking your weight less often can mean that you might discover one day that you've gained a lot of weight without realising it, which could lead you to question why you bothered to slim at all, potentially leading to your heading even further off course.

It's particularly important to weigh yourself after a 'bad' patch (that hen weekend away, that stressed-out week at work where you

> **❝ If you weigh yourself regularly you'll quickly notice if you've gained any weight and can take prompt action to lose it again ❞**

lived on full-fat cappuccinos and cake). From personal experience, even though I usually return from cocktail-fuelled holidays feeling less than virtuous and suspecting I've put on at least half a stone (3.2kg), I'm invariably

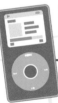

WHAT TO DO IF YOU GAIN MORE THAN 5LB (2.3KG)

1 Consider the cause – start filling in your *Adore Yourself Slim* Travel Journal again (see page 148).

2 Analyse how and why your healthy habits have changed.

3 Deal with the gain by asking yourself what strategies worked for you before.

4 Review the possible solutions and then decide on which one(s) to use.

pleasantly surprised to find that I've only gained a pound or two (making my trainers the first thing I pack so I can go running while abroad really does help, as does having lost the taste for fatty and unhealthy foods), which is a great spur to return to super-healthy eating sooner rather than later. When you know exactly where you stand, you can regroup and recommit. On the other hand, when you're blindly guessing what damage you've done, you're far more likely to squeeze in a few more days of dodgy eating as you wallow in guilt and self-loathing. Don't! Confess to your sins quickly, then repent!

HYPNOTISE YOURSELF SLIM – FOR LIFE! TRACK 5

To help you maintain your new healthy mindset, I'd like you to now start listening to Track 5 (Stay Slim) on your hypnosis CD at least once, and preferably twice, a day. This track is designed to continue to inspire you, encourage you and applaud you, so that the lifestyle changes you've made will last a lifetime. Once you feel completely confident that all the changes you've made are permanent, you can listen to this track less often, but do play it at least occasionally (it's your Secret Slimming Tool, after all, but will only work if you actually use it once in a while) to help you continue adoring yourself slim.

MAINTAINING YOUR DREAM WEIGHT THE *ADORE YOURSELF SLIM* WAY

Now that you want to stabilise at your new healthier weight, you need to get into energy balance – where the calories you consume are in balance with the energy you burn. Because you've lost weight, your daily calorie/energy needs will be a bit lower than they were at your higher weight because there's less of you to burn energy. After losing a realistic 5–10% of your weight (see page 49), you may feel that you're happy with your new weight and want to maintain it long term. Or, if you were very overweight to start with, and would like to lose more weight for your health's sake, this *Adore Yourself Slim* Stay Slim Plan can help you spend some time getting used to living at your new weight before moving on to lose even more.

Because you haven't been following a quick-fix diet plan or extreme exercise programme but making small, sustainable lifestyle changes, there shouldn't be a dramatic change to what you do next, as you've been establishing the habits, skills and mindset you need to maintain your weight. If your weight has already naturally stabilised, then as long as you're sticking to The Basic Healthy Eating Guidelines (see the box, right) there isn't much that you need to change. If you've been continuing to lose weight up until the time you decide to stabilise, then you can eat a bit more. This is best done by adding in an extra daily serving of nutritious food, little by little (see above right), until your weight stabilises.

THE *ADORE YOURSELF SLIM* STAY SLIM PLAN

1 Add in one food serving of about 100–130 calories every day for a week (see Possible Foods To Add In, opposite, for ideas). Use them to make a bigger meal or have them as a snack.

2 Check what's happened to your weight at the end of the week. If it has stabilised, there's no need to add any more servings. If it hasn't, have a second extra serving every day for another week, repeating this process until your weight has stabilised. You may also decide to 'bank' a few days of extra servings for a meal out. Check your weight regularly (and your waist measurement or how your fitted clothes feel, if you like) and aim to keep it within a 4–7lb (2–3kg) range.

3 While the Stay Slim Plan suggests adding in a few foods that you may not have eaten for a while in a step-wise way, you'll notice that not every possible option is

> ### THE BASIC HEALTHY EATING GUIDELINES
> ■ Eat three regular meals plus two planned snacks a day.
> ■ Include a lean/low-fat Protein/or Dairy serving and vegetables, salad or fruit at every meal.
> ■ Include at least three servings of Nutritious Carbohydrates daily.
> ■ Limit deep-fried, high-fat and sugary foods (and drinks).
> ■ Stick to the recommended daily limits of alcohol, and have at least six to eight sugarless drinks daily (and don't forget to drink plenty of water).

listed, as that list would be very long! The plan focuses on making the majority of your food choices nutrient dense, but that doesn't mean you can never eat pâté or pizza again. Remember the advice regarding eating out and Sanity Savers: if there's anything you like eating that's not on the plan, then by all means have some, but limit yourself to an occasional small portion. However, use the foods on the *Adore Yourself Slim* Eating Plan/Stay Slim Plan to make up the majority of what you eat.

4 Don't forget to keep up your reward system by giving yourself non-food-related treats after every two to three months that you've managed to maintain your weight, and when you've got back on track after a gain (see page 47 for ideas).

5 You will inevitably have ups and downs, so please don't ever beat yourself up. Forgive, forget and refocus. You can't be, nor need be, perfect all the time. It's a great idea to meet regularly with the members of your Goal Group and to continue to fill in your *Adore Yourself Slim* Travel Journal. And be sure to use any of the other motivational tools you've found helpful in this book, such as the hypnosis CD.

6 Most importantly, keep congratulating yourself on what you've achieved! Keep smiling at your new double-chin-free face in the mirror and keep buying clothes that best display your fabulous new figure. Revel in being responsible for, and in charge of, your weight! By doing this, you're certain to find that this newfound self-belief will enhance other areas of your life, too.

▶ **POSSIBLE FOODS TO ADD IN**

- 2 extra Fruit servings
- 1 extra Nutritious Carbohydrates serving
- 1 extra Dairy serving
- 2 level tbsp (30g) pesto
- ½ avocado
- 1 palmful of nuts or seeds
- Chocolate/snack food (up to 130 calories)
- 150g (5½oz) pot low-fat rice pudding or low-fat custard
- 60g (2¼oz)/1 scoop ice cream
- 200ml (7fl oz) glass of fruit juice or fruit smoothie
- 125ml (4fl oz) glass of wine or 285ml (½ pint)/1 small bottle of beer or cider/25-35ml (1-1¼fl oz) spirits plus low-calorie mixer (see page 68 for recommended limits)

'WE DID IT, SO CAN YOU!'

I've been on some ridiculous diets in my time and it took me over 30 years to finally realise that I didn't have to torture myself with the latest fad diet but needed instead to make sustainable lifestyle changes with a view to the long term. Having adopted a healthy-eating plan and reached my goal weight over three years ago, I've maintained a healthy weight ever since. I focus on eating foods with a high nutritional value and avoid 'empty' calories. I weigh myself once a week on Sundays and if I've gained a little weight I deal with it right away – it's a lot easier to lose 2lb (0.9kg) than 2st (12.7kg). I don't believe in dieting, which implies short-term deprivation; a healthy lifestyle requires mindful eating, but the focus is on living not calorie counting. For me maintenance is not black and white (it's hot pink!). There's not a lengthy list of do's and don'ts, just one key principle: if you put on a little weight one week, lose it the next.

Sharon Dermody, 45, teacher, Paris

'Having been a card-carrying member of the yo-yo weight loss/ diet roundabout, I'm proud to say that, three years on from losing 3st (19kg) mainly through walking, I still have my weight under control (and I've not been near a diet). The way I've stayed slim is to continue going walking whenever possible, and by being really careful about everything I put in my mouth. Think about it. That double custard Danish you're about to devour. What is it really going to do for you? Sure, it looks like heaven on a plate and it will taste divine for the 120 seconds it takes to eat, but it'll probably make you feel hungrier later and nutritionally it'll do absolutely nothing for you. I don't believe in labelling foods as "good" or "bad", just in making informed choices. As delicious as pastries and cakes are, I now limit them to once-in-a-blue-moon treats, as I realise they don't do me any nutritional favours at all.'

Liz Dallas, 37, research analyst, London

'I've maintained my weight by not falling into the trap of thinking "I've exercised today, so I've earned this bar of chocolate, crisps or biscuit." I try to think of naughty foody treats as cancelling out the good I've achieved with the exercise. When I feel the need to "reward" myself, I make sure it's a healthy treat like a piece of fruit – or better still, when I feel I deserve a pat on the back for staying a healthy weight, I treat myself to a manicure, a massage, a new piece of clothing or a haircut.'

**Jo Penny, 34,
researcher, London**

'I was overweight when I left university (I'm 5ft 5in/1.65m and weighed 11st 7lb/73kg). Some of the weight came off due to the post-university change in lifestyle – less beer, fewer lie-ins and fewer tuna-mayonnaise toasties – and I dropped to about 10st (63.5kg), where I plateaued for several years. Then I discovered triathlon. Finding a sport I was passionate about meant I became more toned, my weight fell gradually and naturally to 9st (57.2kg) and the pounds have never gone back on again. And I'm not talking about excessive amounts of exercise: I train three or four times a week for no more than an hour. My weight has stayed the same for six years now.'

**Lisa Buckingham, 32,
journalist and author, London**

'Although I always cook balanced, healthy meals, my biggest problem has always been portion sizes. If I don't feel full and satisfied, then I want more! So every evening meal that I cook, I dish up my husband's dinner, put a lunch-sized portion in an airtight container for the next day and then serve up the rest on my plate. This reduces the amount I eat and means there's none left in the pan for seconds. If I was to carefully measure out the correct amounts to start with, then it wouldn't look like much in the pan and I'd start thinking that I'm depriving myself. I never want to think I'm missing out on anything, so gaining a tasty and free lunch the next day is an added bonus.'

**Vanessa Aminian, 33,
graphic designer, Stockport**

'One thing I do to maintain my weight if I've had a small gain is to write down everything I eat, and weigh myself every week. I find it harder to snack on cheese or to justify pouring myself that relaxing waiting-for-my-husband-to-come-home-from-work glass of wine when I'm forced to record my misdeeds! Another thing that helps is to wear trousers with a fitted waistband (no elastic and no leggings). This prevents me from deceiving myself that my clothes are all lovely and loose fitting and happily concluding that I haven't gained any weight.'

**Barbara Johnson, 36,
lawyer, Singapore**

'Having previously lost a lot of weight and then, unable to endure the deprivation, put it back on again (plus the requisite extra 1st 6lb/9kg), this is what I've learned: by all means eat healthily and exercise, but do give yourself treats and don't sacrifice things you don't want to stay off for ever. To that end, I have small sweet treats fairly regularly and desserts (mmm, cheesecake!) from time to time. I've still lost lots of weight (albeit more slowly), but this time it feels absolutely sustainable. Life is good.'

**Linda Jackson, 53,
training coordinator, Winnipeg, Canada**

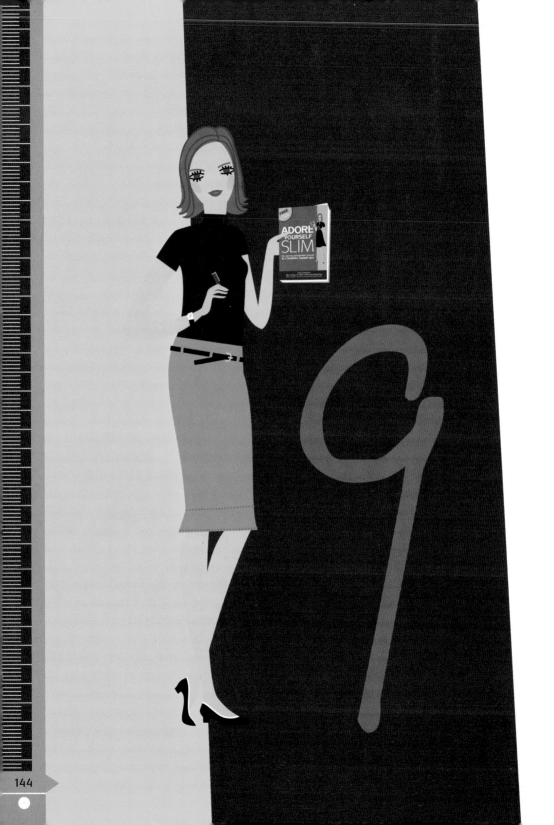

ADORE
YOURSELF
SLIM

Chapter 9

WRITE yourself SLIM

'I can live for two months on a good compliment,' Mark Twain once wrote, which is why this chapter includes a page where you can note down all those lovely things everyone's been saying about the new you. Whenever you feel tempted to plunder the pick 'n' mix or go bonkers for biscuits, simply turn to page 147 for an instant dose of encouragement. There's also a three-month diary, The *Adore Yourself Slim* Travel Journal, where you can jot down all the healthy food you eat, and every energising exercise and motivating hypnosis session you do. So get out that pen and start scribbling your way to success…

KEEP A COUNT OF YOUR COMPLIMENTS

Sadly, most dieters are so beset by low self-esteem that they fail to realise that they can look good, or even great, right this very instant. They think they'll only deserve praise when they're at their goal weight. But they're wrong. This book is all about loving yourself during the journey of getting slim, not just once you've got to Destination Dream Weight, so I'd like you to start seeing compliments as little signposts that confirm you're heading in the right direction. That's why it's vital to take them very seriously indeed. Start by filling them in on the page opposite.

DIARISE IT AND DOUBLE YOUR RESULTS

On the page overleaf, you'll find The *Adore Yourself Slim* Travel Journal, which is also a vitally important part of this programme (a study[1] has shown that people who kept a diary at least five days a week *doubled* their weight loss compared to those who didn't). There's space to record everything you do, along with your daily rewards, the things you're grateful for (so you get a little feel-good boost every day), your Random Acts of Kindness and any slip-ups you can learn from. Note that there's a slot both for your current target weight (perhaps losing that first ½st/3.2kg, then small, step-by-step targets) and also space for your Destination Dream Weight – the weight you ultimately want to get to. It may feel like a bit of a drag to fill in at first, but trust me, it really is worth the effort!

> 66 **The happiness of life is made up of minute fractions – the little, soon-forgotten charities of a kiss or a smile, a kind look or heartfelt compliment** 99
> *Samuel Taylor Coleridge*

LISA'S COMPLIMENTS COLLECTION

DATE	NAME	COMPLIMENT
25/4	Kelly M	'Your face looks different – it's somehow thinner' (day 5)
14/5	Alex	'Are you wearing trousers a couple of sizes too big for you?'
31/7	Laura	'Hello super-skinny Lisa!'
3/10	Cynthia	'You've lost sooo much weight' via email after seeing my Médoc Marathon photo (right)
4/11	Bridget	'Wow, you look amazing!'

MY FAVOURITE COMPLIMENTS COLLECTION

DATE	NAME	COMPLIMENT
28/3	Nicolais	You have an amazing figure
28/5	WM	You look Hot tonight

THE *ADORE YOURSELF SLIM* TRAVEL JOURNAL

DATE	BREAKFAST	SNACK	LUNCH	SNACK	DINNER

Non-alcoholic drinks   Alcoholic drinks   Hypnosis AM/PM

Sneaky Workout   Cardio workout   Resistance workout

Weight/BMI   Current target weight   Daily reward

DATE	BREAKFAST	SNACK	LUNCH	SNACK	DINNER

Non-alcoholic drinks   Alcoholic drinks   Hypnosis AM/PM

Sneaky Workout   Cardio workout   Resistance workout

Weight/BMI   Current target weight   Daily reward

DATE	BREAKFAST	SNACK	LUNCH	SNACK	DINNER

Non-alcoholic drinks   Alcoholic drinks   Hypnosis AM/PM

Sneaky Workout   Cardio workout   Resistance workout

Weight/BMI   Current target weight   Daily reward

DATE	BREAKFAST	SNACK	LUNCH	SNACK	DINNER

Non-alcoholic drinks   Alcoholic drinks   Hypnosis AM/PM

Sneaky Workout   Cardio workout   Resistance workout

Weight/BMI   Current target weight   Daily reward

DATE	BREAKFAST	SNACK	LUNCH	SNACK	DINNER

Non-alcoholic drinks _____ Alcoholic drinks _____ Hypnosis AM/PM

Sneaky Workout _____ Cardio workout _____ Resistance workout

Weight/BMI _____ Current target weight _____ Daily reward

DATE	BREAKFAST	SNACK	LUNCH	SNACK	DINNER

Non-alcoholic drinks _____ Alcoholic drinks _____ Hypnosis AM/PM

Sneaky Workout _____ Cardio workout _____ Resistance workout

Weight/BMI _____ Current target weight _____ Daily reward

DATE	BREAKFAST	SNACK	LUNCH	SNACK	DINNER

Non-alcoholic drinks _____ Alcoholic drinks _____ Hypnosis AM/PM

Sneaky Workout _____ Cardio workout _____ Resistance workout

Weight/BMI _____ Current target weight _____ Daily reward

Weight lost so far _____ Destination Dream Weight _____

This week I'm so happy that _____

_____

Random Acts of Kindness performed _____

Any slip-ups I can learn from? _____

DATE	BREAKFAST	SNACK	LUNCH	SNACK	DINNER

Non-alcoholic drinks   Alcoholic drinks   Hypnosis AM/PM
Sneaky Workout   Cardio workout   Resistance workout
Weight/BMI   Current target weight   Daily reward

DATE	BREAKFAST	SNACK	LUNCH	SNACK	DINNER

Non-alcoholic drinks   Alcoholic drinks   Hypnosis AM/PM
Sneaky Workout   Cardio workout   Resistance workout
Weight/BMI   Current target weight   Daily reward

DATE	BREAKFAST	SNACK	LUNCH	SNACK	DINNER

Non-alcoholic drinks   Alcoholic drinks   Hypnosis AM/PM
Sneaky Workout   Cardio workout   Resistance workout
Weight/BMI   Current target weight   Daily reward

DATE	BREAKFAST	SNACK	LUNCH	SNACK	DINNER

Non-alcoholic drinks   Alcoholic drinks   Hypnosis AM/PM
Sneaky Workout   Cardio workout   Resistance workout
Weight/BMI   Current target weight   Daily reward

DATE	BREAKFAST	SNACK	LUNCH	SNACK	DINNER

Non-alcoholic drinks   Alcoholic drinks   Hypnosis AM/PM

Sneaky Workout   Cardio workout   Resistance workout

Weight/BMI   Current target weight   Daily reward

DATE	BREAKFAST	SNACK	LUNCH	SNACK	DINNER

Non-alcoholic drinks   Alcoholic drinks   Hypnosis AM/PM

Sneaky Workout   Cardio workout   Resistance workout

Weight/BMI   Current target weight   Daily reward

DATE	BREAKFAST	SNACK	LUNCH	SNACK	DINNER

Non-alcoholic drinks   Alcoholic drinks   Hypnosis AM/PM

Sneaky Workout   Cardio workout   Resistance workout

Weight/BMI   Current target weight   Daily reward

Weight lost so far   Destination Dream Weight

This week I'm so happy that

Random Acts of Kindness performed

Any slip-ups I can learn from?

DATE	BREAKFAST	SNACK	LUNCH	SNACK	DINNER

Non-alcoholic drinks   Alcoholic drinks   Hypnosis AM/PM

Sneaky Workout   Cardio workout   Resistance workout

Weight/BMI   Current target weight   Daily reward

DATE	BREAKFAST	SNACK	LUNCH	SNACK	DINNER

Non-alcoholic drinks   Alcoholic drinks   Hypnosis AM/PM

Sneaky Workout   Cardio workout   Resistance workout

Weight/BMI   Current target weight   Daily reward

DATE	BREAKFAST	SNACK	LUNCH	SNACK	DINNER

Non-alcoholic drinks   Alcoholic drinks   Hypnosis AM/PM

Sneaky Workout   Cardio workout   Resistance workout

Weight/BMI   Current target weight   Daily reward

DATE	BREAKFAST	SNACK	LUNCH	SNACK	DINNER

Non-alcoholic drinks   Alcoholic drinks   Hypnosis AM/PM

Sneaky Workout   Cardio workout   Resistance workout

Weight/BMI   Current target weight   Daily reward

DATE	BREAKFAST	SNACK	LUNCH	SNACK	DINNER

Non-alcoholic drinks _____ Alcoholic drinks _____ Hypnosis AM/PM

Sneaky Workout _____ Cardio workout _____ Resistance workout

Weight/BMI _____ Current target weight _____ Daily reward

DATE	BREAKFAST	SNACK	LUNCH	SNACK	DINNER

Non-alcoholic drinks _____ Alcoholic drinks _____ Hypnosis AM/PM

Sneaky Workout _____ Cardio workout _____ Resistance workout

Weight/BMI _____ Current target weight _____ Daily reward

DATE	BREAKFAST	SNACK	LUNCH	SNACK	DINNER

Non-alcoholic drinks _____ Alcoholic drinks _____ Hypnosis AM/PM

Sneaky Workout _____ Cardio workout _____ Resistance workout

Weight/BMI _____ Current target weight _____ Daily reward

Weight lost so far _____ Destination Dream Weight _____

This week I'm so happy that _____

_____

Random Acts of Kindness performed _____

Any slip-ups I can learn from? _____

_____

DATE	BREAKFAST	SNACK	LUNCH	SNACK	DINNER

Non-alcoholic drinks   Alcoholic drinks   Hypnosis AM/PM

Sneaky Workout   Cardio workout   Resistance workout

Weight/BMI   Current target weight   Daily reward

DATE	BREAKFAST	SNACK	LUNCH	SNACK	DINNER

Non-alcoholic drinks   Alcoholic drinks   Hypnosis AM/PM

Sneaky Workout   Cardio workout   Resistance workout

Weight/BMI   Current target weight   Daily reward

DATE	BREAKFAST	SNACK	LUNCH	SNACK	DINNER

Non-alcoholic drinks   Alcoholic drinks   Hypnosis AM/PM

Sneaky Workout   Cardio workout   Resistance workout

Weight/BMI   Current target weight   Daily reward

DATE	BREAKFAST	SNACK	LUNCH	SNACK	DINNER

Non-alcoholic drinks   Alcoholic drinks   Hypnosis AM/PM

Sneaky Workout   Cardio workout   Resistance workout

Weight/BMI   Current target weight   Daily reward

DATE	BREAKFAST	SNACK	LUNCH	SNACK	DINNER

Non-alcoholic drinks   Alcoholic drinks   Hypnosis AM/PM

Sneaky Workout   Cardio workout   Resistance workout

Weight/BMI   Current target weight   Daily reward

DATE	BREAKFAST	SNACK	LUNCH	SNACK	DINNER

Non-alcoholic drinks   Alcoholic drinks   Hypnosis AM/PM

Sneaky Workout   Cardio workout   Resistance workout

Weight/BMI   Current target weight   Daily reward

DATE	BREAKFAST	SNACK	LUNCH	SNACK	DINNER

Non-alcoholic drinks   Alcoholic drinks   Hypnosis AM/PM

Sneaky Workout   Cardio workout   Resistance workout

Weight/BMI   Current target weight   Daily reward

Weight lost so far   Destination Dream Weight

This week I'm so happy that

Random Acts of Kindness performed

Any slip-ups I can learn from?

DATE	BREAKFAST	SNACK	LUNCH	SNACK	DINNER

Non-alcoholic drinks   Alcoholic drinks   Hypnosis AM/PM

Sneaky Workout   Cardio workout   Resistance workout

Weight/BMI   Current target weight   Daily reward

DATE	BREAKFAST	SNACK	LUNCH	SNACK	DINNER

Non-alcoholic drinks   Alcoholic drinks   Hypnosis AM/PM

Sneaky Workout   Cardio workout   Resistance workout

Weight/BMI   Current target weight   Daily reward

DATE	BREAKFAST	SNACK	LUNCH	SNACK	DINNER

Non-alcoholic drinks   Alcoholic drinks   Hypnosis AM/PM

Sneaky Workout   Cardio workout   Resistance workout

Weight/BMI   Current target weight   Daily reward

DATE	BREAKFAST	SNACK	LUNCH	SNACK	DINNER

Non-alcoholic drinks   Alcoholic drinks   Hypnosis AM/PM

Sneaky Workout   Cardio workout   Resistance workout

Weight/BMI   Current target weight   Daily reward

DATE	BREAKFAST	SNACK	LUNCH	SNACK	DINNER

Non-alcoholic drinks   Alcoholic drinks   Hypnosis AM/PM

Sneaky Workout   Cardio workout   Resistance workout

Weight/BMI   Current target weight   Daily reward

DATE	BREAKFAST	SNACK	LUNCH	SNACK	DINNER

Non-alcoholic drinks   Alcoholic drinks   Hypnosis AM/PM

Sneaky Workout   Cardio workout   Resistance workout

Weight/BMI   Current target weight   Daily reward

DATE	BREAKFAST	SNACK	LUNCH	SNACK	DINNER

Non-alcoholic drinks   Alcoholic drinks   Hypnosis AM/PM

Sneaky Workout   Cardio workout   Resistance workout

Weight/BMI   Current target weight   Daily reward

Weight lost so far   Destination Dream Weight

This week I'm so happy that

Random Acts of Kindness performed

Any slip-ups I can learn from?

DATE	BREAKFAST	SNACK	LUNCH	SNACK	DINNER

Non-alcoholic drinks   Alcoholic drinks   Hypnosis AM/PM

Sneaky Workout   Cardio workout   Resistance workout

Weight/BMI   Current target weight   Daily reward

DATE	BREAKFAST	SNACK	LUNCH	SNACK	DINNER

Non-alcoholic drinks   Alcoholic drinks   Hypnosis AM/PM

Sneaky Workout   Cardio workout   Resistance workout

Weight/BMI   Current target weight   Daily reward

DATE	BREAKFAST	SNACK	LUNCH	SNACK	DINNER

Non-alcoholic drinks   Alcoholic drinks   Hypnosis AM/PM

Sneaky Workout   Cardio workout   Resistance workout

Weight/BMI   Current target weight   Daily reward

DATE	BREAKFAST	SNACK	LUNCH	SNACK	DINNER

Non-alcoholic drinks   Alcoholic drinks   Hypnosis AM/PM

Sneaky Workout   Cardio workout   Resistance workout

Weight/BMI   Current target weight   Daily reward

DATE	BREAKFAST	SNACK	LUNCH	SNACK	DINNER

Non-alcoholic drinks   Alcoholic drinks   Hypnosis AM/PM

Sneaky Workout   Cardio workout   Resistance workout

Weight/BMI   Current target weight   Daily reward

DATE	BREAKFAST	SNACK	LUNCH	SNACK	DINNER

Non-alcoholic drinks   Alcoholic drinks   Hypnosis AM/PM

Sneaky Workout   Cardio workout   Resistance workout

Weight/BMI   Current target weight   Daily reward

DATE	BREAKFAST	SNACK	LUNCH	SNACK	DINNER

Non-alcoholic drinks   Alcoholic drinks   Hypnosis AM/PM

Sneaky Workout   Cardio workout   Resistance workout

Weight/BMI   Current target weight   Daily reward

Weight lost so far   Destination Dream Weight

This week I'm so happy that

Random Acts of Kindness performed

Any slip-ups I can learn from?

DATE	BREAKFAST	SNACK	LUNCH	SNACK	DINNER

Non-alcoholic drinks   Alcoholic drinks   Hypnosis AM/PM

Sneaky Workout   Cardio workout   Resistance workout

Weight/BMI   Current target weight   Daily reward

DATE	BREAKFAST	SNACK	LUNCH	SNACK	DINNER

Non-alcoholic drinks   Alcoholic drinks   Hypnosis AM/PM

Sneaky Workout   Cardio workout   Resistance workout

Weight/BMI   Current target weight   Daily reward

DATE	BREAKFAST	SNACK	LUNCH	SNACK	DINNER

Non-alcoholic drinks   Alcoholic drinks   Hypnosis AM/PM

Sneaky Workout   Cardio workout   Resistance workout

Weight/BMI   Current target weight   Daily reward

DATE	BREAKFAST	SNACK	LUNCH	SNACK	DINNER

Non-alcoholic drinks   Alcoholic drinks   Hypnosis AM/PM

Sneaky Workout   Cardio workout   Resistance workout

Weight/BMI   Current target weight   Daily reward

DATE	BREAKFAST	SNACK	LUNCH	SNACK	DINNER

Non-alcoholic drinks   Alcoholic drinks   Hypnosis AM/PM

Sneaky Workout   Cardio workout   Resistance workout

Weight/BMI   Current target weight   Daily reward

DATE	BREAKFAST	SNACK	LUNCH	SNACK	DINNER

Non-alcoholic drinks   Alcoholic drinks   Hypnosis AM/PM

Sneaky Workout   Cardio workout   Resistance workout

Weight/BMI   Current target weight   Daily reward

DATE	BREAKFAST	SNACK	LUNCH	SNACK	DINNER

Non-alcoholic drinks   Alcoholic drinks   Hypnosis AM/PM

Sneaky Workout   Cardio workout   Resistance workout

Weight/BMI   Current target weight   Daily reward

Weight lost so far   Destination Dream Weight

This week I'm so happy that

Random Acts of Kindness performed

Any slip-ups I can learn from?

DATE	BREAKFAST	SNACK	LUNCH	SNACK	DINNER

Non-alcoholic drinks   Alcoholic drinks   Hypnosis AM/PM

Sneaky Workout   Cardio workout   Resistance workout

Weight/BMI   Current target weight   Daily reward

DATE	BREAKFAST	SNACK	LUNCH	SNACK	DINNER

Non-alcoholic drinks   Alcoholic drinks   Hypnosis AM/PM

Sneaky Workout   Cardio workout   Resistance workout

Weight/BMI   Current target weight   Daily reward

DATE	BREAKFAST	SNACK	LUNCH	SNACK	DINNER

Non-alcoholic drinks   Alcoholic drinks   Hypnosis AM/PM

Sneaky Workout   Cardio workout   Resistance workout

Weight/BMI   Current target weight   Daily reward

DATE	BREAKFAST	SNACK	LUNCH	SNACK	DINNER

Non-alcoholic drinks   Alcoholic drinks   Hypnosis AM/PM

Sneaky Workout   Cardio workout   Resistance workout

Weight/BMI   Current target weight   Daily reward

DATE	BREAKFAST	SNACK	LUNCH	SNACK	DINNER

Non-alcoholic drinks   Alcoholic drinks   Hypnosis AM/PM

Sneaky Workout   Cardio workout   Resistance workout

Weight/BMI   Current target weight   Daily reward

DATE	BREAKFAST	SNACK	LUNCH	SNACK	DINNER

Non-alcoholic drinks   Alcoholic drinks   Hypnosis AM/PM

Sneaky Workout   Cardio workout   Resistance workout

Weight/BMI   Current target weight   Daily reward

DATE	BREAKFAST	SNACK	LUNCH	SNACK	DINNER

Non-alcoholic drinks   Alcoholic drinks   Hypnosis AM/PM

Sneaky Workout   Cardio workout   Resistance workout

Weight/BMI   Current target weight   Daily reward

Weight lost so far   Destination Dream Weight

This week I'm so happy that

Random Acts of Kindness performed

Any slip-ups I can learn from?

DATE	BREAKFAST	SNACK	LUNCH	SNACK	DINNER

Non-alcoholic drinks   Alcoholic drinks   Hypnosis AM/PM
Sneaky Workout   Cardio workout   Resistance workout
Weight/BMI   Current target weight   Daily reward

DATE	BREAKFAST	SNACK	LUNCH	SNACK	DINNER

Non-alcoholic drinks   Alcoholic drinks   Hypnosis AM/PM
Sneaky Workout   Cardio workout   Resistance workout
Weight/BMI   Current target weight   Daily reward

DATE	BREAKFAST	SNACK	LUNCH	SNACK	DINNER

Non-alcoholic drinks   Alcoholic drinks   Hypnosis AM/PM
Sneaky Workout   Cardio workout   Resistance workout
Weight/BMI   Current target weight   Daily reward

DATE	BREAKFAST	SNACK	LUNCH	SNACK	DINNER

Non-alcoholic drinks   Alcoholic drinks   Hypnosis AM/PM
Sneaky Workout   Cardio workout   Resistance workout
Weight/BMI   Current target weight   Daily reward

DATE	BREAKFAST	SNACK	LUNCH	SNACK	DINNER

Non-alcoholic drinks   Alcoholic drinks   Hypnosis AM/PM

Sneaky Workout   Cardio workout   Resistance workout

Weight/BMI   Current target weight   Daily reward

DATE	BREAKFAST	SNACK	LUNCH	SNACK	DINNER

Non-alcoholic drinks   Alcoholic drinks   Hypnosis AM/PM

Sneaky Workout   Cardio workout   Resistance workout

Weight/BMI   Current target weight   Daily reward

DATE	BREAKFAST	SNACK	LUNCH	SNACK	DINNER

Non-alcoholic drinks   Alcoholic drinks   Hypnosis AM/PM

Sneaky Workout   Cardio workout   Resistance workout

Weight/BMI   Current target weight   Daily reward

Weight lost so far   Destination Dream Weight

This week I'm so happy that

Random Acts of Kindness performed

Any slip-ups I can learn from?

DATE	BREAKFAST	SNACK	LUNCH	SNACK	DINNER

Non-alcoholic drinks   Alcoholic drinks   Hypnosis AM/PM

Sneaky Workout   Cardio workout   Resistance workout

Weight/BMI   Current target weight   Daily reward

DATE	BREAKFAST	SNACK	LUNCH	SNACK	DINNER

Non-alcoholic drinks   Alcoholic drinks   Hypnosis AM/PM

Sneaky Workout   Cardio workout   Resistance workout

Weight/BMI   Current target weight   Daily reward

DATE	BREAKFAST	SNACK	LUNCH	SNACK	DINNER

Non-alcoholic drinks   Alcoholic drinks   Hypnosis AM/PM

Sneaky Workout   Cardio workout   Resistance workout

Weight/BMI   Current target weight   Daily reward

DATE	BREAKFAST	SNACK	LUNCH	SNACK	DINNER

Non-alcoholic drinks   Alcoholic drinks   Hypnosis AM/PM

Sneaky Workout   Cardio workout   Resistance workout

Weight/BMI   Current target weight   Daily reward

DATE	BREAKFAST	SNACK	LUNCH	SNACK	DINNER

Non-alcoholic drinks   Alcoholic drinks   Hypnosis AM/PM

Sneaky Workout   Cardio workout   Resistance workout

Weight/BMI   Current target weight   Daily reward

DATE	BREAKFAST	SNACK	LUNCH	SNACK	DINNER

Non-alcoholic drinks   Alcoholic drinks   Hypnosis AM/PM

Sneaky Workout   Cardio workout   Resistance workout

Weight/BMI   Current target weight   Daily reward

DATE	BREAKFAST	SNACK	LUNCH	SNACK	DINNER

Non-alcoholic drinks   Alcoholic drinks   Hypnosis AM/PM

Sneaky Workout   Cardio workout   Resistance workout

Weight/BMI   Current target weight   Daily reward

Weight lost so far   Destination Dream Weight

This week I'm so happy that

Random Acts of Kindness performed

Any slip-ups I can learn from?

DATE	BREAKFAST	SNACK	LUNCH	SNACK	DINNER

Non-alcoholic drinks | Alcoholic drinks | Hypnosis AM/PM

Sneaky Workout | Cardio Workout | Resistance workout

Weight/BMI | Current target weight | Daily reward

DATE	BREAKFAST	SNACK	LUNCH	SNACK	DINNER

Non-alcoholic drinks | Alcoholic drinks | Hypnosis AM/PM

Sneaky Workout | Cardio Workout | Resistance workout

Weight/BMI | Current target weight | Daily reward

DATE	BREAKFAST	SNACK	LUNCH	SNACK	DINNER

Non-alcoholic drinks | Alcoholic drinks | Hypnosis AM/PM

Sneaky Workout | Cardio Workout | Resistance workout

Weight/BMI | Current target weight | Daily reward

DATE	BREAKFAST	SNACK	LUNCH	SNACK	DINNER

Non-alcoholic drinks | Alcoholic drinks | Hypnosis AM/PM

Sneaky Workout | Cardio Workout | Resistance workout

Weight/BMI | Current target weight | Daily reward

DATE	BREAKFAST	SNACK	LUNCH	SNACK	DINNER

Non-alcoholic drinks   Alcoholic drinks   Hypnosis AM/PM

Sneaky Workout   Cardio workout   Resistance workout

Weight/BMI   Current target weight   Daily reward

DATE	BREAKFAST	SNACK	LUNCH	SNACK	DINNER

Non-alcoholic drinks   Alcoholic drinks   Hypnosis AM/PM

Sneaky Workout   Cardio workout   Resistance workout

Weight/BMI   Current target weight   Daily reward

DATE	BREAKFAST	SNACK	LUNCH	SNACK	DINNER

Non-alcoholic drinks   Alcoholic drinks   Hypnosis AM/PM

Sneaky Workout   Cardio workout   Resistance workout

Weight/BMI   Current target weight   Daily reward

Weight lost so far   Destination Dream Weight

This week I'm so happy that

Random Acts of Kindness performed

Any slip-ups I can learn from?

DATE	BREAKFAST	SNACK	LUNCH	SNACK	DINNER

Non-alcoholic drinks　　　　　　　　　Alcoholic drinks　　　　　　　　　Hypnosis AM/PM

Sneaky Workout　　　　　　　Cardio workout　　　　　　　Resistance workout

Weight/BMI　　　　　　Current target weight　　　　　Daily reward

DATE	BREAKFAST	SNACK	LUNCH	SNACK	DINNER

Non-alcoholic drinks　　　　　　　　　Alcoholic drinks　　　　　　　　　Hypnosis AM/PM

Sneaky Workout　　　　　　　Cardio workout　　　　　　　Resistance workout

Weight/BMI　　　　　　Current target weight　　　　　Daily reward

DATE	BREAKFAST	SNACK	LUNCH	SNACK	DINNER

Non-alcoholic drinks　　　　　　　　　Alcoholic drinks　　　　　　　　　Hypnosis AM/PM

Sneaky Workout　　　　　　　Cardio workout　　　　　　　Resistance workout

Weight/BMI　　　　　　Current target weight　　　　　Daily reward

DATE	BREAKFAST	SNACK	LUNCH	SNACK	DINNER

Non-alcoholic drinks　　　　　　　　　Alcoholic drinks　　　　　　　　　Hypnosis AM/PM

Sneaky Workout　　　　　　　Cardio workout　　　　　　　Resistance workout

Weight/BMI　　　　　　Current target weight　　　　　Daily reward

DATE	BREAKFAST	SNACK	LUNCH	SNACK	DINNER

Non-alcoholic drinks   Alcoholic drinks   Hypnosis AM/PM

Sneaky Workout   Cardio workout   Resistance workout

Weight/BMI   Current target weight   Daily reward

DATE	BREAKFAST	SNACK	LUNCH	SNACK	DINNER

Non-alcoholic drinks   Alcoholic drinks   Hypnosis AM/PM

Sneaky Workout   Cardio workout   Resistance workout

Weight/BMI   Current target weight   Daily reward

DATE	BREAKFAST	SNACK	LUNCH	SNACK	DINNER

Non-alcoholic drinks   Alcoholic drinks   Hypnosis AM/PM

Sneaky Workout   Cardio workout   Resistance workout

Weight/BMI   Current target weight   Daily reward

Weight lost so far   Destination Dream Weight

This week I'm so happy that

Random Acts of Kindness performed

Any slip-ups I can learn from?

REFERENCES

CHAPTER 1

1 Cochrane, G; Friesen, J (1986). Hypnotherapy in weight-loss treatment. *J Consult Clin Psychol*, 54: 489-492

2 Bolocofsky, DN; Spinler, D; Coulthard-Morris, L (1985). Effectiveness of hypnosis as an adjunct to behavioural weight management. *J Clin Psychol*, 41: 35-41

CHAPTER 3

1 Jung, RT (1997). Obesity as a disease. *Br Med Bull*, 53: 307-321

CHAPTER 4

1 Slavin, J (2004). Wholegrains and human health. *Nutr Res Rev*, 17(1): 99-110

2 Van Baak, MA et al. Weight-loss maintenance on *ad libitum* diets varying in protein content and glycaemic index: first results of the DIOGENES highly controlled shop-based intervention. Abstract presented at the ECO 2008, Geneva. http://www.diogenes-eu.org

3 Clifton, PM et al (2008). Long-term effects of a high-protein weight-loss diet. *AJCN*, 87(1): 23-29

4 NICE. Obesity: the prevention, identification, assessment and management of overweight and obesity in adults and children. NICE clinical guideline no 43. London, NICE; 2006 www.nice.org.uk/guidance/CG43

5 Timlin, MT; Pereira, MA (2007). Breakfast frequency and quality in the etiology of adult obesity and chronic diseases. *Nutr Rev*, 65: 268-281

6 Hirsch, AR et al (2007). Effect of television viewing on sensory-specific satiety: are Leno and Letterman obesogenic? 89th Annual Meeting Endocrine Society Abstract Book, 175

7 Kokkinos, A et al (2010). Eating slowly increases the postprandial response of the anorexigenic gut hormones, peptide YY and glucagon-like peptide-1. *J Clin Endocrinol Metab*, 95(1): 333-337

8 Westenhoefer, J (2001). The therapeutic challenge: behavioural changes for long-term weight maintenance. *Int J Obes Relat Metab Disord*, 25(Suppl 1): S85-S88

9 Paddon-Jones, D et al (2008). Protein, weight management and satiety. *AJCN*, 87(5): 1558S-1561S

10 Zemel, MB et al (2004). Calcium and dairy acceleration of weight and fat loss during energy restriction in obese adults. *Obes Res*, 12(4): 582-590

11 Yao, M et al (2001). Dietary energy density and weight regulation. *Nutr Rev*, 59(8): 247-258

12 Shai, I; Stampfer, MJ (2008). Weight-loss diets – can you keep it off? *AJCN*, 88(5): 1185-1186

12 Sacks, FM et al (2009). Comparison of weight-loss diets with different compositions of fat, protein and carbohydrates. *N Engl J Med*, 360: 859-873

13 Rolls, BJ et al (2006). Reductions in portion size and energy density of foods are additive and lead to sustained decreases in energy intake. *AJCN*, 83(1): 11-17

14 Flood, JE; Rolls, BJ (2007). Soup preloads in a variety of forms reduce meal energy intake. *Appetite*, 49(3): 626-634

15 Bertrais, S et al (2001). Consumption of soup and nutritional intake in French adults: consequences for nutritional status. *JHND*, 14(2): 121-128

16 Hursel, R; Westerterp-Plantenga, MS (2010). Thermogenic ingredients and bodyweight regulation. *IJO*, 34: 659-669

17 Phung, OJ et al (2010). Effect of green tea catechins with or without caffeine on anthropometric measures: a systematic review and meta-analysis. *AJCN*, 91(1): 73-81

18 Ahuja, KDK et al (2006). Effects of chilli

consumption on postprandial glucose, insulin and energy metabolism. *AJCN*, 84(1): 63-69

19 Bourdon, I et al (2001). Beans, as a source of dietary fibre, increase cholecystokinin and apolipoprotein B48 response to test meals in men. *J Nutr*, 131: 1485-1490

20 Vander Wal, JS (2008). Egg breakfast enhances weight loss. *IJO*, 32(10): 1545-1551

21 Rolls, BJ et al (2004). Salad and satiety: energy density and portion size of a first-course salad affect energy intake at lunch. *J Am Diet Assoc*, 104(10): 1570-1576

22 Maruyama, K et al (2008). The joint impact on being overweight of self-reported behaviours of eating quickly and eating until full: cross-sectional survey. *BMJ*, 337: a2002

23 Roberts, C et al (2007). The effects of stress on bodyweight: biological and psychological predictors of change in BMI. *Obesity*, 15: 3045-3055

24 Leproult, R; Van Cauter, E (2010). Role of sleep and sleep loss in hormonal release and metabolism. *Endocr Dev*, 17: 11-21

25 Chandon, P; Wansink, B (2007). The biasing health halos of fast-food restaurant health claims: lower calorie estimates and higher side-dish consumption intentions. *J Consum Res*, 34: 301-314

26 Holt, SH et al (1995). A satiety index of common foods. *Eur J Clin Nutr*, 49(9): 675-690

CHAPTER 5

1 Wing, RR; Phelan, S (2005). Long-term weight loss maintenance. *AJCN*, 82(1): 222S-225S

2 Franco, OH; De Laet, C; Peeters, A; Jonker, J; Mackenbach, J; Nusselder, W (2005). Effects of physical activity on life expectancy with cardiovascular disease. *Arch Intern Med*, 165: 2355-2360

3 Bravata, DM; Smith-Spangler, C; Sundaram, V et al (2007). Using pedometers to increase physical activity and improve health: a systematic review. *JAMA*, 298(19): 2296-2304

4 Kraemer, WJ et al (1999). Influence of exercise training on physiological and performance changes with weight loss in men. *Med Sci Sports Exerc*, 31(9): 1320-1329

5 Bryner, RW; Toffle, RC; Ullrish IH; Yeater, RA (1997). The effects of exercise intensity on body composition, weight loss and dietary composition in women. *J Am Col Nutr*, 16(1): 68-73

6 Tremblay, A; Simoneau, JA; Bouchard, C (1994). Impact of exercise intensity on body fatness and skeletal muscle metabolism. *Metabolism*, 43(7): 814-818

7 Stone, MH; Fleck, SJ; Triplett, NT; Kraemer, WJ (1991). Health- and performance-related potential of resistance training. *Sports Med*, 11(4): 210-231

8 Francis, P; Davis, J. Research conducted at the San Diego State University Biomechanics Lab

CHAPTER 8

1 National Weight Control Registry research findings. www.nwcr.ws/Research

1 Kayman, S et al (1990). Maintenance and relapse after weight loss in women: behavioural aspects. *AJCN*, 52: 800-807

1 Westenhoefer, J (2001). The therapeutic challenge: behavioural changes for long-term weight maintenance. *Int J Obes Relat Metab Disord*, 25(Suppl 1): S85-S88

CHAPTER 9

1 Hollis, J et al (2008). Weight loss during the intensive intervention phase of the weight-loss maintenance trial. *Am J Prev Med*, 35(2): 118-126

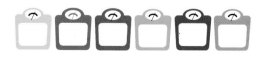

THANK YOU TO…

… Francine Lawrence for believing in this book right from the very outset and for her invaluable advice and considerable creative contribution.

… everyone at Simon & Schuster who worked so hard to create this book: Ami Richards, Nicky Hill, Lorraine Jerram, Geoff Fennell, Katherine Thornton and Prudence Ivey.

… dietitian Lyndel Costain (www. lyndelcostain.co.uk) who encouraged me to make my eating plan as healthy as it could be. The wealth of professional experience she contributed to *Adore Yourself Slim* has ensured that all the advice in this book is clinically sound, evidence based and, most importantly, infinitely practical.

… Coach Bronek (www.coachbronek.com) who made me believe that the impossible was possible in the gym.

… personal trainer Sarah Maxwell (www.sarahmaxwell.co.uk) who despite her million-miles-an-hour lifestyle always found time to reply to my emails immediately and is a living example of someone who practises what they preach.

… Jayne Ellis (www.reinventmystyle.com) who made a huge contribution to the style section and made Pat and I fall in love with fashion when she styled us for our shoot.

… Angela Ryan (www.angelaryan.co.uk) whose design brought this book to life. Her professionalism, creative flair and sense of humour made her a joy to work with.

… Maxim Savva (http://maximsavva.com), whose delightful illustrations never cease to make me smile.

… Sarah Owen, Loren Jackson, Jo Richardson, Graham Williams, Delia Roberts and Bridget Robinson whose untiring enthusiasm and wonderfully insightful editing have immeasurably improved this book.

… Davy Nougarede, David Roper and Pete Smith at Heavy Entertainment who produced the hypnosis CD.

… Rod Williams, who composed the wonderfully relaxing music on the CD.

… Peter Mabbutt, Sjanie Hugo Wurlitzer and Janice Champion for their hypnotherapy input.

… Jackie Graveney, Angie Govender, Loren Jackson, Penny Warren and Tracey Beresford for their very useful comments on my book proposal.

… Bridget Robinson, my friend and slimming buddy, who continues to live the dream and help me achieve mine.

… all my wonderful patients who've shared their weight-loss journeys with me, in particular those who so generously agreed to be featured in this book: Pat Ivory, Kirsty Brown and Carmen Nel. And to all the women from around the world who sent me their best slimming tips, only a few of which I could include in this book.

… photographer Claire Richardson (www. clairerichardson.com) and her assistant Ellie Laycock for their awe-inspiring attention to detail while shooting this book's photos.

… food stylist Lizzie Harris (07976 434224) who made sure the photographs did justice to how appetising healthy food can be.

… Freire Wright who so kindly let us take over her Hammersmith home for our shoot.

… Roland Hale and Sasha Krisiunaite Solveigh at Toni & Guy, Soho (www.toniandguy.com), who styled my and Pat Ivory's hair; hairstylist Robert Woodward who cut and coloured Pat's hair; and Jackie Planson (make-up).

… Emma Sherman at Rush Hair, Moorgate (020 7871 0353), for her advice on hair.

… David Pistorius and Kevin Stewart.

… Nikki Campbell, Don Oliver, Braam